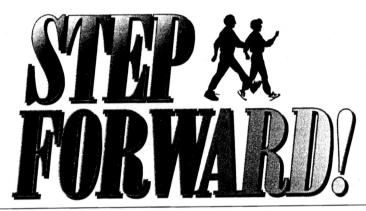

# STEP FORWARD!

## A Christian 12-Step Program to Lose Weight—*and Keep It Off!*

### UNIT 2

### PARTICIPANT'S WORKBOOK

JULIE MORRIS

Abingdon Press

Step Forward:
A Christian 12-Step Programto Lose Weight—*and Keep It Off!*
Unit 2 Participant's Workbook

Julie Morris

Copyright 1998 by Abingdon Press

ISBN 0-687-08756-2

Note: The publisher and/or author are not responsible for failure on the part of any individual or group of individuals to lose weight or to maintain weight loss on the Step Forward program. Consult a physician before beginning any weight loss program.

Art on pages 10, 14, 18, 27, 32, 37, 43, 48, 54, 61, 68, and 72 are by Dolf Seeds. Instructional design and graphics for Victory List and Food Journal on pages 75—76 by Katherine Coleman.

---

**Note:** The Step Forward Twelve Steps are modeled after the Twelve Steps of Alcoholics Anonymous:
1. We admitted that we were powerless over alcohol—that our lives had become unmanageable.
2. Came to believe that a Power grater than ourselves could restore us to sanity.
3. Made a decision to turn our will and our lives over to the care of God as we understood Him.
4. Made a searching and fearless moral inventory of ourselves.
5. Admitted to God, to ourselves, and to another human being the exact nature of our wrongs.
6. We were entirely ready to have God remove all these defects of character.
7. Humbly asked Him to remove our shortcomings.
8. Made a list of all persons we had harmed, and became willing to make amends to them all.
9. Made direct amends to such people wherever possible, except when to do so would injure them or others.
10. Continued to take personal inventory and when we were wrong promptly admitted it.
11. Sought through prayer and meditation to improve our conscious contact with God as we understood Him, praying only for knowledge of His will for us and the power to carry that out.
12. Having had a spiritual awakening as the result of these steps, we tried to carry this message to alcoholics, and to practice these principles in all of our affairs.

The Twelve Steps are reprinted with permission of Alcoholics Anonymous World Services, Inc. Permission to reprint and adapt the Twelve Steps does not mean that AA has reviewed or approved the contents of this publication, nor that AA agrees with the views expressed herein. AA is a program of recovery from alcoholism. Use of the Twelve Steps in connection with programs that are patterned after AA but that address other problems does not imply otherwise.

# Contents

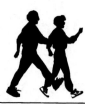

# STEP FORWARD'S TWELVE STEPS

**Step 1**   We admitted that we were powerless over food and that our lives had become unmanageable.

**Step 2**   Came to believe that God, through Jesus Christ, could restore us to sanity.

**Step 3**   Made a decision to turn our will and our lives over to the care of God through Jesus Christ.

**Step 4**   Made a searching and fearless moral inventory of ourselves.

**Step 5**   Admitted to God, to ourselves, and to another human being the exact nature of our wrongs.

**Step 6**   Were entirely ready to have God remove all these defects of character.

**Step 7**   Humbly asked God to remove our shortcomings.

**Step 8**   Made a list of all persons we have harmed, and became willing to make amends to them all.

**Step 9**   Made direct amends to such people wherever possible, except when to do so would injure them or others.

**Step 10**   Continued to take personal inventory and when we were wrong, promptly admitted it.

**Step 11**   Sought through prayer and meditation to improve our conscious contact with God through Jesus Christ, praying for knowledge of his will for us and for the power to carry that out.

**Step 12**   Having had a spiritual awakening, tried to carry this message to compulsive overeaters and to practice these principles in all our affairs.

By first recognizing our need for God's help (Step 1) and then focusing on God's ability (Step 2), we come to a point at which we are able to make a decision to surrender our will and every aspect of our lives (including our eating) to God's care (Step 3). Then we learn to recognize and surrender our weaknesses, sins, and broken relationships to God (Steps 4–9). Maintenance steps teach us to continue to walk closely with God on a daily basis, to rely on God's grace, and to share what he is teaching us with others (Steps 10–12).

As we work the Twelve Steps presented in the sessions of the four units, share insights from the Bible relating to the steps, and use the Stepping Stones of the Step Forward program, we learn how to deal with our problems and our feelings rather than eating over them. We learn to cast our cares on the Lord and not the refrigerator.

**Session 1:**

# Why Do I Need a Life Preserver?

**GUIDING PRINCIPLE:** *I can learn to trust God all the time.*

## APPLICATION QUESTION

*Review the lies that we discussed during the last session: lies about worth, security, approval, blame, and shame. Which lie affects your life the most? Why?*

Share what you wrote on the following from Ratha's *Search For Significance* (Robert S. McGee, Rapha Resources, 1985): "I am deeply loved, fully pleasing, totally forgiven, accepted and complete in Christ."

## PRINCIPLES FROM THE WORD

Read one of the meditations you wrote on last week's assigned Scripture passages as it relates to living with the truth instead of with lies.

## STEPPING STONE SURVEY

Share a step forward! How did one of the Stepping Stones help you this week?

## SPIRITUAL FOCUS

In preparation for beginning Step 3 this week, we will review Steps 1 and 2.

*Write Step 1 and Step 2 in the blanks below.*

Step 1:_____

_____

Step 2:_____

_____

*Answer and discuss the following questions:*

**1. How have I taken Step 1?**

_____

_____

**2. How have I taken Step 2?**

_____

_____

**3. How has my eating been insane? (This is also the Physical Focus.)**

_____

_____

**Step 3:** Made a decision to turn our will and our lives over to the care of God through Jesus Christ.

*Write Step 3 in this space, thinking about the words as you write them.*

_____

_____

_____

In order to surrender our will and our lives, we must first begin with trust. We trust because we have found that we are powerless. We have no choice but to reach out for help unless we want to remain in the same unmanageable lifestyle. We trust an all–powerful God who can restore us to sanity. We trust an all–loving God who wants to restore us to sanity. We trust an all–knowing God who understands how to restore us to sanity. How do we trust? We make a decision!

**According to Step 1, why do we trust?** _____

_____

**According to Step 2, whom do we trust?** _____

_____

**According to Step 3, how do we trust?** _____

_____

## An Analogy on Trust

Decide how the first three steps apply to the following analogy, taken from Rapha's *12 Step Program for Overcoming Eating Disorders* (Robert S. McGee, Wm. Drew Mountcastle):

"You have fallen overboard and someone throws you a life preserver. What actions would be involved with each step?"

*Write the correct step number in the blank in front of each action.*

**Step** _____ You see the life preserver, realize that you need it and that it can help you right now.

**Step** _____ You put it on and keep it on!

**Step** _____ You recognize that you may drown and call for help.

*"Why is it so hard to leave your life preserver on?"*
In other words, why is it so hard to turn our eating disorder over to God and to leave it there?

*Take notes as the group discusses each of the following excuses.*

• There must be an easier way than wearing this thing and floating in the water!

_____

_____

• Maybe if I cling to someone or something else, I will be more secure. After all, how can I be sure that this thing will float forever?

_____

_____

• Why did I get on that boat anyway? I wish I hadn't fallen overboard.

_____

_____

• Others keep telling me I shouldn't wear the life preserver and that something else works better.

_____

_____

• This thing is uncomfortable sometimes and restricting.

_____

_____

• I might feel better if I took it off. It gets in the way of my swimming.

_____

_____

### How does this life preserver work?

• I don't have to understand it, just wear it.
• I have a choice. I can do the dog paddle instead of putting it on and just take my chances.
• After I put it on, the one who threw it draws me closer to himself, brings me to safety, and encourages me to stay in the boat until we get to shore.
• There may come a time that it's too late to put it on. **What does this mean?**

_____

_____

_____

### A Quotation on Trust

Think about this quotation from Jerry Bridges' *Trusting God*: "We must choose, by an act of our will, to trust God in major and minor difficulties. We can do this regardless of how we may feel, because we know that God is sovereign, wise, and loving."

*Do you trust God in all difficulties, both major and minor? What helps you to see God as sovereign? as wise? as loving?*

_____

_____

_____

_____

### A Willingness to Trust

*By working program, how can we trust God?*

• *By working the steps.* John 15:5c—"Apart from me (Jesus said) you can do nothing."

*How does this verse relate to working the first three steps?*

We can trust God more as we work the steps because we learn to recognize that . . .

1. We can't!
2. God can!
3. We'll let him!

• **By letting go and letting God.** *Psalm 46:10a*—"Be still, and know that I am God."

*What can you let go of? Circle the examples that apply to you.*

Compulsive overeating!

Trying to do things without God's help.

Excusing myself and blaming others.

Trying to change others and take God's job.

Demanding my own way.

*What are some indications that you are letting go? Circle the responses that apply to you.*

I am eating right.

I am not as frustrated by other people because I am working my own program.

I am not as angry or worried.

I want to spend more time with God.

I am able to relax more, and my life isn't so unmanageable.

• **By acting "as if . . ."** *Mark 9:24b*—"I do believe; help me overcome my unbelief!"

*When the man asking for a miracle in this Scripture admitted his lack of complete faith, what was Jesus' reaction?*

_____

_____

*How can I act "as if" I truly trust God? List three or four ways.*

_____

_____

_____

_____

## PHYSICAL FOCUS

This is covered in the Spiritual Focus section under the question, "How has my eating been insane?"

# PRACTICING THE PRINCIPLES
(Homework)

1. Do you believe that you have taken Steps 1 and 2? Why?

2. List specific things that you can do to learn to trust God more. Put one or two of them on your Victory List.

3. Memorize verses from this lesson:

   • *John 15:5c*—Apart from me (Jesus said) you can do nothing.

   • *Psalm 46:10a*—Be still, and know that I am God.

   • *Mark 9:24b*—I do believe; help me overcome my unbelief!

4. Meditate on the following verses about learning to trust God:
   • Psalm 20:7
   • Deuteronomy 9:23
   • Proverbs 3:5-6
   • Psalm 16:1-2
   • Psalm 46:1

*Julie's Thoughts to Munch On*

Staying on track is so much easier than getting on track.

This thing sure gets in the way!

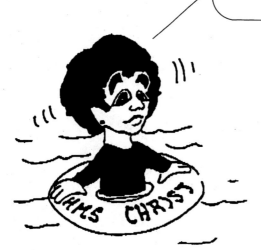

**Session 2:**

# Why Is It So Hard to Surrender?

**GUIDING PRINCIPLE:** *I can surrender to God so I'll quit stumbling so much.*

## APPLICATION QUESTION

*Last week we discussed learning how to trust God more. What things are you doing to learn how to do this? What would you like to try?*

*Write Steps 1, 2, and 3 in the blanks below:*

**Step 1:** _____

_____

**Step 2:** _____

_____

**Step 3:** Made a decision to _____ to the care of _____

## PRINCIPLES FROM THE WORD

Read one of the meditations you wrote on last week's assigned Scripture passages as it relates to learning to trust God.

## STEPPING STONE SURVEY

*Write the sentence that helps us remember the Stepping Stones (there are nine of them):*

_____

*List all the Stepping Stones and suggest ways to use each one:*

_____

_____

_____

_____

_____

_____

_____

_____

_____

## SPIRITUAL FOCUS

This week's Spiritual Focus centers on identifying and dealing with the thoughts, feelings, and circumstances that keep us from letting go and letting God.

Following is a list of Stumbling Blocks that can stand in the way of us surrendering completely to God. **Put a checkmark beside the ones that apply to your own struggles.** Share your biggest Stumbling Block and suggest something that could help you overcome that obstacle (a Blockbuster). A Blockbuster could be a Bible verse, a positive thought, or one of the nine Stepping Stones. Take notes during the class discussion under each Stumbling Block of things that might help you to let go and let God.

❏ Unable to let go. Thoughts keep coming back.

_____

❏ Thinking I can manipulate God by good deeds into doing what I want him to do.

_____

❏ Too busy to pray.

_____

❏ Unwilling to have his way instead of my own.

_____

❏ Belief that I can (or should) do it better alone.

_____

❏ False guilt—"bothering God" with my small problems.

_____

❏ Feeling of unworthiness to ask for his help (again).

_____

❏ Too distracted with worries to remember he's there.

_____

❏ Incomplete Second Step: not understanding God's sovereignty.

_____

❏ Others need me too much for me to take time for myself.

_____

❏ Turning to food instead of dealing with problems.

_____

❏ Belief that God doesn't care.

_____

❏ Thought that I can't be God's child until I'm "good enough."

_____

❏ Idea that I can always do it tomorrow.

_____

❏ Unwillingness to change or extreme fear of it.

_____

❏ Living a life of regret—believing the lie: "It's too late."

_____


## PHYSICAL FOCUS

*How can I surrender my food cravings to God and overcome them permanently? By cooperating with God as he changes my desires!*

• Recognize foods and ways of eating that trigger my cravings and determine that the few minutes of pleasure they bring just aren't worth the pain that the cravings cause.

| Some possible trigger foods | Some trigger ways of eating |
|---|---|
| 1. | |
| 2. | |
| 3. | |
| 4. | |
| 5. | |

• Don't complain.

_____

• Don't fantasize.

_____

• Be thankful.

_____

• Be consistent.

_____

• Act "as if."

_____

_____

## PRACTICING THE PRINCIPLES
(Homework)

1. Briefly review each Stumbling Block and the Blockbusters for each one discussed in class.

2. Write on three of the Stumbling Blocks and how they hinder your taking the Third Step completely.

3. Write a prayer surrendering your food cravings to God. Pray for willingness to do what God is leading you to do to cooperate with him so you can get rid of your cravings.

4. Meditate on the following verses. Find the Blockbuster in each one:
   • Psalm 119:165
   • Matthew 16:23
   • 1 Corinthians 1:22–24
   • Proverbs 3:21–26
   • Jude 24

*Julie's Thoughts to Munch On*

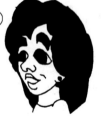

*God doesn't play tug-of-war with me. When I get what I demand, I get consequences I deserve.*

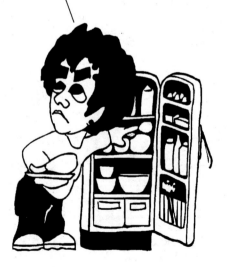

*How can a refrigerator be a stumbling block?*

**Session 3:**

# How Can I Trust When It Hurts?

**GUIDING PRINCIPLE:** *I can trust God to use the adversity in my life.*

## APPLICATION QUESTION

*Give steps forward that you are making in surrendering a particular problem to God—for example, a relationship, weakness, fear, bad habit, old hurt, or regret. Try not to repeat an answer that already has been mentioned.*

## PRINCIPLES FROM THE WORD

Share one of the meditations you wrote on last week's assigned Scripture passages as it relates to surrendering to God.

## STEPPING STONE SURVEY

This session's Stepping Stone focus is on Accountability. Step Forward encourages members to choose an accountability partner or coach to help them stay on track. Answer the questions below as a review of using a partner or coach to stay accountable:

*What are some desirable qualities in an accountability partner or a coach?*

_____

_____

_____

_____

*What are the advantages of being an accountability partner and/or coach?*

_____

_____

_____

_____

*What can you do if you aren't working with one now?*

_____

_____

_____

## SPIRITUAL FOCUS

This week's discussion continues to focus on Step 3—surrender—by looking at the prerequisite to surrender: trusting God.

*When is it hardest to trust God?*

_____

_____

_____

**What are the advantages of adversity?** The book *Trusting God*, by Jerry Bridges (Nave Press), offers the following suggestions (words listed below, in bold). Be prepared to take turns reading a Bible verse and discussing how it relates to Bridges' thoughts on why God allows adversity in our lives.

### Pruning

*1 Peter 4:1b-2*—He who has suffered in his body is done with sin. As a result, he does not live the rest of his earthly life for evil human desires, but rather for the will of God.

_____

_____

### Holiness

*Job 2:4b-5*—Satan replied, "A man will give all he has for his own life. But stretch out your hand and strike his flesh and bones, and he will surely curse you to your face."

_____

_____

### Dependence

*Psalm 18:2*—The Lord is my rock, my fortress and my deliverer; my God is my rock, in whom I take refuge. He is my shield and the horn of my salvation, my stronghold.

_____

_____

### Perseverance

*James 1:2-4*—Consider it pure joy, my brothers, whenever you face trials of many kinds, because you know that the testing of your faith develops perseverance. Perseverance must finish its work so that you may be mature and complete, not lacking anything.

_____

_____

**Service**

*2 Corinthians 1:3-4*—Praise be to the God and Father of our Lord Jesus Christ the father of compassion and the God of all comfort who comforts us in all our troubles so that we can comfort those in any trouble with the comfort we ourselves have received from God.

_____

_____

**Fellowship**

*2 Corinthians 1:7b*—We know that just as you share in our sufferings, so also you share in our comfort.

_____

_____

**Relationship with God**

*Psalm 34:18*—The Lord is close to the broken hearted and saves those who are crushed in spirit.

_____

_____

*What must we do to profit from adversity? In other words:*

*• What attitude must we have when submitting to God?*

_____

_____

*• What is our text as we take the Lab Course of painful situations?*

_____

_____

*• Why must we remember our pain?*

_____

_____

## PHYSICAL FOCUS

**As a review, fill in the calorie content for the following items. You will find the answers in the back of this workbook.**

| Item | Calories |
|------|----------|
| Meat, 1 ounce, lean | _____ |
| Meat, 1 ounce, medium | _____ |
| Meat, 1 ounce, marbled | _____ |

Bread, 1 serving _____

Fruit, 1 serving _____

Vegetable, 1 serving _____

Milk, 8 ounces, skim _____

Milk, 8 ounces, 2 percent _____

Milk, 8 ounces, 4 percent _____

Mayonnaise, 1 tablespoon _____

Peanut butter, 1 tablespoon _____

Egg, large _____

Vegetable oil, 1 tablespoon _____

Cheese, 1 ounce _____ (approx.)

## PRACTICING THE PRINCIPLES
(Homework)

1. When did you experience the most adversity in your life?

2. Refer to the section on the advantages of adversities. How did you see growth during this time?

3. How has your eating disorder encouraged spiritual growth?

4. Memorize the facts you have forgotten about calories.

5. Meditate on the following verses. List further benefits of adversity as you find them in the verses.
   - 2 Corinthians 4:8–10
   - 2 Corinthians 4:16–18
   - 2 Corinthians 6:3–10
   - Hebrews 12:7–11
   - 2 Corinthians 1:8–10

***Julie's Thoughts to Munch On:***

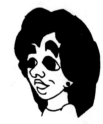

*I don't know what the future holds, but I know who holds the future.*

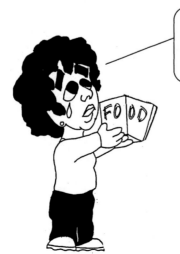

*I won't say "Why me?" Now I'll say, "What would you have me learn?"*

**Session 4:**

# Who, Me . . . Worry?

**GUIDING PRINCIPLE:** *I can overcome my worries.*

## APPLICATION QUESTION

*How did God use the time of your life when you were dealing with the most adversity? What good things came out of your pain? Be prepared to discuss your answers.*

*How has your eating disorder encouraged emotional and/or spiritual growth? Put a checkmark beside the answers that apply to your own personal experience.*

❏ I have learned that I had to depend on God, even for small things.

❏ I have learned to be more disciplined, for example, having daily quiet time.

❏ I have met lots of really nice people in Step Forward and have learned to be honest with them and not wear a mask.

❏ I have learned that God could do the impossible in me when I cooperate.

❏ I have learned to live one day at a time and persevere.

❏ I have learned that God uses my weaknesses and failures for my good if I turn them over to him.

❏ I have been able to help others with my same problem.

❏ I am seeing miracles of restoration occur in my life, not only physically, but emotionally and spiritually as well.

# PRINCIPLES FROM THE WORD

Share one of the meditations that you wrote on last week's Bible verses.

Take turns reading the following verses and the related advantages that we discover when we trust God during times of adversity.

### 2 Corinthians 4:8–10
- I learn how to persevere.
- I learn that God's promises are really true.
- I experience God's presence. He seems closer to me.
- I have the opportunity to reflect Jesus' qualities, such as bearing up to adversity without crumbling.

### 2 Corinthians 4:16–18
- I feel God's restoration.
- I build up treasures in heaven and look forward to going.
- I learn to have a heavenly perspective.
- I can leave earthly ties behind more easily.

### 2 Corinthians 6:3–10
- I am a good witness to others.
- Others notice me and hear my testimony.
- I am able to practice what I preach.
- I know that it is God working in me.

### Hebrews 12:7–11
- I am not spoiled and am well–trained.
- I respect God more.
- I become holier through discipline.
- I have more peace in my life.

### 2 Corinthians 1:8–10
- I learn how to endure pain with God's help.
- I realize how short life is.
- I recognize my powerlessness.
- I see God's miracles of deliverance!

### Can you think of some other advantages of adversity?

_____

_____

_____

# STEPPING STONE SURVEY

Prayer is an important Stepping Stone. And part of prayer—the often-forgotten half—is listening. Today's Stepping Stone discussion will focus on listening.

*How can I listen?*

_____

_____

*In what ways does God "speak" to me?*

_____

_____

# SPIRITUAL FOCUS

*Write the first three steps below.*

Step 1: _____

_____

Step 2: _____

_____

Step 3: _____

_____

# Worry

This week's Spiritual Focus deals with worry, and how it relates to the Third Step.

*Why discuss worry with the Third Step?*

_____

_____

Read this Scripture from 1 John 4:18 (Living Bible):

> "We need have no fear of someone who loves us perfectly. His perfect love eliminates all dread of what he might do to us. If we are afraid it is for fear of what he might do to us and shows that we are not fully convinced that he really loves us."

*According to ti~~~rse, ~~~ ha~~~does worrying show?*

_____

_____

*How can we quit worrying?*

**Step 1:** Admit _____!

**Step 2:** Remember _____!
**Step 3:** I'll _____!

*How can we begin the process of learning how to quit worrying? Take the prescription God prescribes in Philippians 4:4-7:*

> "Rejoice in the Lord always. I will say it again: rejoice! Let your gentleness be evident to all. The Lord is near. Do not be anxious about anything, but in everything by prayer and petition, with thanksgiving, present your requests to God. And the peace of God, which transcends all understanding, will guard your hearts and your mind in Christ Jesus."

Follow those directions carefully. And remember: Praise is the antidote to panic!

*How can I deal with worry?*

• Make a list of your worries.

• Say "The Serenity Prayer" over your list: "God grant me the serenity to accept the things I cannot change, the courage to change the things I can, and the wisdom to know the difference."

• Put an * next to the things you cannot change. Put these things on your Miracle List to pray over daily.

• Make an Action Plan for each item on your list that you can change. (See Week 5 in the first unit if you are a new member, or if you need to review Action Plans.)

  1. Remember, the problem has to be your problem.
  2. The goal must be realistic and involve only your actions.
  3. The actions must be achievable.
  4. Focus on some of God's qualities and promises:

## God's Qualities and Promises

Read through the list of God's qualities and promises this week. Each day choose a verse to meditate on.

**God has all power, wisdom and knowledge.**
   *Daniel 2:20–22*—Praise be to the name of God, for ever and ever; wisdom and power

are his. He changes times and seasons; he sets up kings and deposes them. He gives wisdom to the wise and knowledge to the discerning. He reveals deep and hidden things; he knows what lies in darkness and light dwells with him.

**God loves me unconditionally as his child because I love Jesus.**

*John 1:12–13*—Yet to all who received him, to those who believed in his name, he gave the right to become children of God. Children born not of natural descent, nor of human decision or a husband's will, but born of God.

**God desires only good things for me, and he has a wonderful plan for my life.**

*Jeremiah 29:11*—"For I know the plans I have for you," declares the Lord, "Plans to prosper you and not to harm you, plans to give you hope and a future."

**God knows everything about me and loves me anyway. He forgives me totally when I sin.**

*1 John 1:9*—If we confess our sins, he is faithful and just and will forgive us our sins and purify us from all unrighteousness.

**Nothing happens to me that does not filter through God's fingers first.**

*Romans 11:36*—For from him and through him and to him are all things. To him be the glory forever! Amen.

**All things do work together for good in my life because I love God and desire his will.**

*Romans 8:28*—And we know that in all things God works for the good of those who love him, who have been called according to his purpose.

**God will never leave me.**

*Romans 8:38–39*—For I am convinced that neither death nor life, neither angels nor demons, neither the present nor the future, nor any powers, neither height nor depth, nor anything else in all creation, will be able to separate us from the love of God that is in Christ Jesus our Lord.

**God will never give me more than I can bear.**

*1 Corinthians 10:13*—God is faithful and he will not let you be tempted beyond what you can bear. But when you are tempted, he will also provide a way out so that you can stand up under it.

**God never commands me to do anything he doesn't enable me to do.**

*Philippians 4:13*—I can do everything through him who gives me strength.

**God writes his law on my heart. (He helps me to want to do his will.)**

*Jeremiah 31:33*—I will put my law in their minds, and write it on their hearts. I will be their God and they will be my people.

**Nothing is impossible for God.**

*Jeremiah 32:27*—"I am the Lord the God of all mankind. Is anything too hard for me?

*Mark 10:27*—Jesus looked at them and said, "With man this is impossible, but not with God; all things are possible with God."

**It's not my ability that God wants to have, but my availability.**

*John 15:4*—Remain in me, and I will remain in you. No branch can bear fruit by itself; it must remain in the vine. Neither can you bear fruit unless you remain in me.

*Psalm 51:17*—The sacrifices of God are a broken spirit; a broken and contrite heart, O God, you will not despise.

**I will not be hungry as I focus on God, but satisfied!**

*Psalm 104:27-28*—These all look to you to give them their food at the proper time. When you give it to them, they gather it up; when you open your hand, they are satisfied with good things.

*Psalm 63:5*—My soul will be satisfied as with the riches of foods; with singing lips my mouth will praise you.

**God always has purpose for my painful circumstances.**

*James 1:2–4*—Consider it pure joy, my brothers whenever you face trials of many kinds, because you know that the testing of your faith develops perseverance. Perseverance must finish its work so that you may be mature and complete, not lacking anything.

**God wants me to rely on him and helps me when I ask him.**

*1 Peter 5:7*—Cast all your anxiety on him because he cares for you.

**If I call out to God, he will answer me. He hears my prayers.**

*Jeremiah 33:3*—Call to me and I will answer you and tell you great and unsearchable things you do not know.

*Jeremiah 29:12*—You will call upon me and come and pray to me, and I will listen to you.

**God made me a new creation in Christ. I will forget the shame of my youth.**

*2 Corinthians 5:17*—Therefore, if anyone is in Christ, he is a new creation; the old has gone; the new has come!

*Isaiah 54:4*—Do not be afraid; you will not suffer shame. Do not fear disgrace; you will not be humiliated. You will forget the shame of your youth.

**After I confess a sin, God "forgets" it ever happened. He doesn't keep a list of my wrongs.**

*Psalm 130:3*—If you, O Lord, kept a record of sins, O Lord, who could stand?

*Psalm 103:12*—As far as the east is from the west, so far has he removed our transgressions from us.

**God teaches me how to solve my problems, but if I overeat in response to problems, I numb my senses so I can't fully respond to his instruction.**

*Proverbs 23:20–21*—Do not join those who drink too much wine or gorge themselves on meat, for drunkards and gluttons become poor, and drowsiness clothes them in rags.

*Psalm 32:8*—I will instruct you and teach you in the way you should go; I will counsel you and watch over you.

**God will abundantly provide for my needs. (He is the one who defines what my needs really are!)**

*2 Corinthians 9:8*—And God is able to make all grace abound to you so that in all things at all times, having all that you need, you will abound in every good work.

*Matthew 6:33*—Seek first his kingdom and his righteousness and all these things (your needs) will be given to you as well.

**God will give me peace in all situations when I focus on him. I can learn to be content in impossible circumstances.**

*Isaiah 26:3*—You will keep in perfect peace him whose mind is steadfast, because he trusts in you.

*Philippians 4:11–13*—I have learned to be content whatever the circumstances. I know what it is to be in need, and I know what it is to have plenty. I have learned the secret of being content in any and every situation, whether well fed or hungry, whether living in plenty or want. I can do everything through him who gives me strength.

**God really understands how I feel.**

*Hebrews 4:15*—For we do not have a high priest who is unable to sympathize with our weaknesses, but we have one who has been tempted in every way, just as we are—yet without sin.

**God is able to keep me from falling. He is my protector and refuge.**

*Jude 24*—To him who is able to keep you from falling and to present you before his glorious presence without fault and with great joy.

*Psalm 32:7*—You are my hiding place; you will protect me from trouble and surround me with songs of deliverance.

**God includes my children in his promises. (They must make their own profession of faith, but God is constantly drawing them to himself!)**

*Isaiah 44:3*—For I will pour water on the thirsty land, and streams on the dry ground; I will pour out my Spirit on your offspring, and my blessing on your descendants.

*Psalm 103:17–18*—From everlasting to everlasting the Lord's love is with those who fear him and his righteousness with their children's children, with those who keep his covenant and remember to obey his precepts.

*Acts 16:31*—Believe in the Lord Jesus, and you will be saved—You and your household.

**I am so precious to God that he knows even the most minute details about me. He thinks about me constantly.**

*Matthew 10:30*—(Jesus said) and even the very hairs of your head are all numbered.

*Isaiah 49:15–16*—Can a mother forget the baby at her breast and have no compassion on the child she has borne? Though she may forget, I will not forget you! See I have engraved you on the palms of my hands.

**I can be absolutely sure I'm going to heaven if I confess Jesus as my personal savior and Lord.**

*Romans 10:9*—If you confess with your mouth, Jesus is Lord, and believe in your heart that God raised him from the dead, you will be saved.

*John 3:16*—For God so loved the world that he gave his one and only son, that whoever believes in him shall not perish but have eternal life.

## PHYSICAL FOCUS

**Ten healthy eating tips are listed below. Circle at least four of them that you will try to incorporate into your menu plan this week.**

1. Rather than drinking juice in the morning, eat a piece of fruit. It takes six oranges to make one large glass of juice, and all the fiber is thrown away.
2. Make a shake in the blender out of skim milk, sugar substitute, a banana, and ice cubes.
3. Make an omelet out of vegetables (mushrooms, onions, and so forth) instead of cheese. Use egg substitutes to save five grams of fat and a bunch of cholesterol.
4. Serve all of your plates from the stove. Never put seconds on the table. That's just asking for trouble. Try to put leftovers in the fridge before the meal.
5. Store food in containers that you can't see through. That way you won't be tempted every time you open the refrigerator door.
6. Reward yourself after you have lost each five pounds. Of course, don't reward yourself with food! Be creative in your rewards: $5 to blow guilt free, going to a movie you haven't had time to see, getting to sleep late one morning. The possibilities are endless.
7. Try new herbs and vinegars. Use them without oil to marinate vegetables and meats.
8. Drink a big glass of water before a meal.
9. Always take something that is on your food plan to a potluck meal.
10. Make fat-free gravy by putting beef or chicken broth in the freezer for an hour in a shallow bowl. Skim the hardened fat off and strain before mixing it with flour. Or use a fat-free gravy packet, or make gravy with a bouillon cube. Imagine that fat on your hips or inside your arteries.

# PRACTICING THE PRINCIPLES

(Homework)

1. Make a list of things you worry about. Put an * next to your top five worries.

2. Choose one verse each day from the list of God's qualities and promises that helps you overcome one of your top five worries. Write a short meditation stating why this verse helps you overcome a specific fear right now.

3. Write a meditation on the following statement and include why it helps you not to be afraid: "I don't know what the future holds, but I know who holds the future!"

4. Choose one verse from this lesson to memorize.

5. Bring your favorite low-fat cooking tip to share next week.

*Julie's Thoughts to Munch On:*

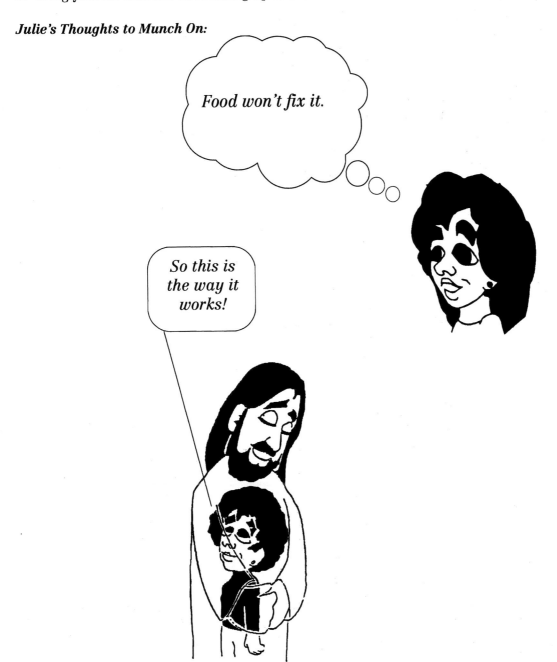

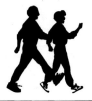

**Session 5:**

# Who Is Trying to Overwhelm Me?

---

**GUIDING PRINCIPLE:** *I can win the spiritual battle if I know whom to fight.*

## APPLICATION QUESTION

*Read what you wrote on the following statement: "I don't know what the future holds, but I know who holds the future!"*

## PRINCIPLES FROM THE WORD

What one thing are you worrying about most? Refer to the verses in the Spiritual Focus section of last week's lesson. Which of these verses helps you to trust God more with this situation? Why? Share your meditation if you wrote one.

## STEPPING STONE SURVEY

This week's Stepping Stone focus in on memorizing. Take a minute to discuss the following sentence:

*Memorizing helps me work program because . . .*

_____

_____

*What are some ways that you can memorize more easily?*

• Make a goal to memorize just three minutes a day, rather than trying to memorize a certain number of Scriptures a week.

• Have a memory section in your notebook. Every time you find a verse that you want to memorize, put it there. Write it neatly in large letters so you can visualize it. Number items in lists included in the verses.

• Divide a sheet of notebook paper in half the long way. Write the Scripture reference on the left side. Write the verse on the right side. On the left, draw a picture of what the verse is saying—whatever helps you visualize the verse.

• Once you've learned a verse, go back and review it from time to time.

*Can you think of other ways to make memorization easier?*

_____

_____

# SPIRITUAL FOCUS

This week's Spiritual Focus is on spiritual warfare.

## What is spiritual warfare?

Read Ephesians 6:12 for the answer: "Our struggle is not against flesh and blood, but against the rulers, against the authorities, against the powers of this dark world and against the spiritual forces of evil in the heavenly realms." According to Ephesians, spiritual warfare is the battle between good and evil forces.

## Why discuss spiritual warfare with the Third Step?

We discuss spiritual warfare with the Third Step because the last thing Satan wants is for us to turn our will and our life over to God's care; he uses all of his tricks to keep us from doing this. We must recognize his tactics to stand firm against him.

## How does Satan tempt us?

Jesus fought his own battle in spiritual warfare when he was tempted by Satan. Read about Jesus' confrontation with Satan in Luke 4:1–13. Some questions on the Scripture passage follow.

1. Jesus, full of the Holy Spirit, returned from the Jordan and was led by the Spirit in the desert.
2. Where for forty days he was tempted by the devil. He ate nothing during those days, and at the end of them he was hungry.
3. The devil said to him, "If you are the son of God, tell this stone to become bread."
4. Jesus answered, "It is written: 'Man does not live on bread alone.' " (Deuteronomy 8:3)
5. The devil led him up to a high place and showed him in an instant all the kingdoms of the world.
6. And he said to him, "I will give you all their authority and splendor, for it has been given to me, and I can give it to anyone I want to.
7. So if you worship me, it will all be yours."
8. Jesus answered, "It is written: 'Worship the Lord your God and serve him only.'" (Deuteronomy 6:13)
9. The devil led him to Jerusalem and had him stand on the highest point of the temple. "If you are the son of God," he said,
10. "Throw yourself down from here. For it is written: 'He will command his angels concerning you to guard you carefully;
11. They will lift you up in their hands, so that you will not strike your foot against a stone.'" (Psalm 91:11,12)
12. Jesus answered, "It says: 'Do not put the Lord your God to the test.'" (Deuteronomy 6:1)
13. When the devil had finished all this tempting, he left him until an opportune time.

**Luke 3 tells us that Jesus was susceptible to temptation for three reasons:**
1. He had just started his ministry.
2. He had just come off a real spiritual high point, his baptism.
3. God said audibly how pleased he was with him. (Do you ever fall into temptation immediately after being praised?)

*What is another reason that Jesus was more susceptible to temptation at that point in his life? (See Luke 4:2.)*

_____

_____

*What was the first thing Satan tempted Jesus with? (See Luke 4:3.)*

_____

_____

*How did Jesus stand up against Satan? (See Luke 4:4.) How can we apply this?*

_____

_____

*What was the second thing he tempted Jesus with? (See Luke 4:6–7.) Do we ever have this temptation?*

_____

_____

*What was his third temptation? How did Satan use Scripture? (See Luke 4:9-13.) Are we ever faced with that?*

_____

_____

### What is Satan like?

Be prepared to take turns reading the following descriptions of Satan, as found in the Bible. Look up the Scripture references this week.

**2 Corinthians 11:14**—Satan masquerades as an angel of light.

**Zechariah 3:1**—Satan is the accuser.

**1 Peter 5:8**—Satan is like a roaring lion looking for someone to devour.

**Revelation 12:9**—Satan is the deceiver.

**John 8:44**—Satan is the father of lies.

**Luke 22:31**—Satan has limited power, only able as God permits him.

**Matthew 25:41**—Satan is doomed.

**James 4:7**—Satan will flee if we resist him.

**Job 1:6–12**—Satan is hostile to anything good.

**Matthew 13:19**—Satan clouds our thinking.

*How do we feel when under attack? Circle the ones that apply to you.*

| | | |
|---|---|---|
| Hopeless | Confused | Defeated |
| Afraid | Angry | Condemned |
| Ashamed | Compulsive | Self-pity |
| Overwhelmed | Nervous | Famished |

*What are some things that make us vulnerable to attack?*

_____

_____

_____

_____

_____

_____

_____

_____

_____

_____

*What are some things we might say if we were under attack?*
Put a checkmark beside the ones you've caught yourself saying or thinking.

❑ "I'll never change, so what's the use?"
❑ "I can't understand why I'm acting this way."
❑ "I'm not even sure that God loves me anymore."
❑ "I just feel overwhelmed with all my problems."
❑ "I hate myself."

## PHYSICAL FOCUS

*Exchange lowfat, no-sugar cooking tips with other members of the class:*

_____

_____

_____

_____

---

**Armaments and Tactics**
How do we stand up against Satan?

Put on the full armor of God and use the tactics he gives us in Ephesians 6:10-18—
- Belt of truth
- Breastplate of righteousness
- Feet fitted with the readiness that comes from the gospel of peace
- Shield of faith
- Helmet of salvation
- Sword of the Spirit
- Pray in the Spirit
- Pray on all occasions
- Pray with all kinds of prayers and requests
- Be alert and always keep on praying for all the saints

---

## PRACTICING THE PRINCIPLES

(Homework)

1. Study Ephesians 6:10–18 this week as it relates to the temptation you face with your eating disorder. Read the entire passage daily and meditate on two of the ten armaments and tactics a day. Write about how each one can help you stand firm in your commitment to eat right.

2. When have you felt at least five of the symptoms of attack at the same time? What happened? What can you do to prepare for the next attack?

3. What are some things that Satan might "whisper in your ear" about food or about your Step Forward program?

4. Write a brief meditation on Romans 8:37 praising God for the victory that is already ours in Christ.

*Julie's Thoughts to Munch On*

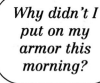

*Why didn't I put on my armor this morning?*

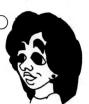

*Why do I want to have foods around that drive me crazy until they're gone?*

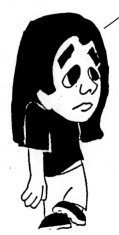

**Session 6:**

# How Can I Win the Battle?

**GUIDING PRINCIPLE:** *I can win the spiritual battle if I learn how to fight.*

## APPLICATION QUESTION

*What are some things that Satan might "whisper in your ear" about food, about your Step Forward program, or about life in general?*

## PRINCIPLES FROM THE WORD

Read your meditation on Romans 8:37 ("... we are more than conquerors through him who loved us"), praising God that the victory is already ours in Christ.

## Armaments and Tactics

*How can each of the ten armaments and tactics mentioned in Ephesians 6:10–18 help us stand firm in our battle for eating right? (This is also the Physical Focus.)*

1. Belt of truth _____

_____

2. Breastplate of righteousness _____

_____

3. Feet ready _____

_____

4. Shield of faith _____

_____

5. Helmet of salvation _____

_____

6. Sword in the Spirit _____

_____

STEP FORWARD—*How Can I Win the Battle?*

7. Pray in the Spirit _____

_____

8. Pray on all occasions _____

_____

9. All kinds of prayers _____

_____

10. Be alert, keep on praying for all the saints _____

_____

### Know the Enemy's Weaknesses

After your leader reads each of the following statements, be prepared to read the accompanying Bible verses.

- **Satan has to flee if we resist him. He is not omnipresent!**
*James 4:7* — "Submit yourselves, then, to God. Resist the devil, and he will flee from you!"

- **Satan has limited power — only able as God permits him. He is not omnipotent!**
*Job 1:10a* — "Satan replied, 'Have you not put a hedge around Job and his household and everything he has . . .?"

- **We have all the power we need through Christ to defeat Satan!**
*2 Corinthians 10:3–5* — "For though we live in the world, we do not wage war as the world does. The weapons we fight with are not the weapons of the world. On the contrary, they have divine power to demolish strongholds. We demolish arguments and every pretension that sets itself up against the knowledge of God and we take captive every thought to make it obedient to Christ."

- **We already knows that Satan is defeated!**
*Romans 16:20* — "The God of peace will soon crush Satan under your feet!"

- **Satan loses when we say the name of Jesus!**
*Romans 10:13* — "Everyone who calls on the name of the Lord will be saved!"

### What three things do we have the power to demolish in our battle with the enemy?

- **Strongholds**—things in my life that I am not surrendering to God.
- **Arguments**—not accepting what God's Word says and holding on to my own ideas, which may be contrary to Scripture.
- **Pretensions**—pretending to surrender to God while clinging to some areas of disobedience, rebellion, or independence.

### What are our "prisoners of war"? How do we make them obedient to Christ?

Our "prisoners of war" are our thoughts. We make them obedient to Christ by recognizing that they are not God's thoughts, recognizing who the author of these thoughts is, and rejecting them. (I cannot empty my mind, so I choose to think about the truth from God's Word instead of Satan's lies.)

## STEPPING STONE SURVEY

*How does each of the Stepping Stones help us when we're under attack? Fill in your answers below.*

*Journaling* _____

_____

*Honesty* _____

_____

*Confidentiality* _____

_____

*Prayer* _____

_____

*Reaching Out* _____

_____

*Food Plan* _____

_____

*Accountability* _____

_____

*Scripture* _____

_____

*Fellowship* _____

_____

## SPIRITUAL FOCUS

How can we win the battle? Know when the battle is coming. Paul describes it in Romans 7:21–25:

> "So I find this law at work: when I want to do good, evil is right there with me. For in my inner being I delight in God's law; but I see another law at work in the members of my body waging war against the law of my mind and making me a prisoner of the law of sin at work within my members. What a wretched man I am! Who will rescue me from this body of death? Thanks be to God it has been done through Jesus Christ our Lord!"

*How does Paul feel?*

_____

_____


*What does Paul remember that helps him to win the battle?*

_____

_____


**Know Satan's strategies and be prepared for them!** Usually he won't encourage us to sin in bold ways, but he will think of more subtle ways to distract us from God. *Circle Satan's strategies that you fall for most often.*

He takes good things (such as helping the homeless) or urgent things (such as errands) and uses them to tempt you away from the eternally important things (such as quiet time, sharing the Lord with your kids).

He takes the Bible and misinterprets it for you. (For example, Matthew 19:29— "Everyone who has left houses or brothers or sisters or father or mother or children or fields for my sake will receive a hundred times as much and will inherit eternal life." Someone misled might say, "Therefore, it's okay for me to divorce my husband so I can share the Lord more.")

He takes empty words that leave Christ out and makes you think they're spiritual because they are poetic.

He makes you think "successful" people who don't love God are happier and are rewarded more than you are.

He portrays almost all Christians on television as wimps or hypocrites and tries to make you ashamed to admit that you are a Christian.

He makes you feel guilty if you do something for yourself, like take time for your program.

He keeps hammering away at you, repeating the same lie until you accept it as your own thought.

He comes at you with problems from several different directions at once so you think you don't know where to turn.

He comes at you when you least expect it (for example, after a big victory).

He encourages you to focus on food, other people, your weaknesses, your circumstances, and anything else that will take your focus off of the Lord.

He makes you think that you are too busy to work program (such as to pray, eat right, attend meetings, journal, and reach out to help others).

He entices you with small acts of disobedience and helps you to rationalize them.

***Battle Plan***
See pages 77 and 78 in the back of this workbook.

## PHYSICAL FOCUS

This week's Physical Focus was covered in the "Principles From the Word" section.

## PRACTICING THE PRINCIPLES
(Homework)

1. Practice using the Battle Plan on pages 77 and 78. (Note: If you are not feeling overwhelmed at this time, write only items 5–9.)

2. Memorize 2 Corinthians 10:5.

3. Write a Third Step prayer turning your will and your life over to God's care using the following:

   "Everything I have comes from you, O Lord. I am open to receive it. I face this day and all of life knowing that you will supply all of my needs."

4. Meditate on the following verses as they relate to the victory that is ours in Christ.
   - 1 John 4:4
   - Psalm 27:1–5
   - 1 Corinthians 15:58
   - Romans 10:13
   - Psalm 34:7

***Julie's Thoughts to Munch On***

*When I want to work program least, I need to work it most.*

*I'm surrounded!*

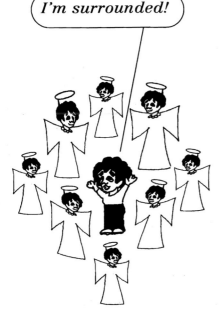

## Session 7:

# Why Should I Look Back When I Want to Step Forward?

---

**GUIDING PRINCIPLE:** *I can grow up if I inventory my childhood.*

## APPLICATION QUESTION

*Name a time since starting program that you have been overwhelmed. Do you think you were under attack? How did you use your program to help you stand firm in your faith?*

## PRINCIPLES FROM THE WORD

Share the Third Step prayer you wrote with the rest of the class. See the one below for an example of how a Third Step might be written.

> *Father, I have tried to surrender my will and my life to you, but I grab back the control so often. I forget that you are in charge and that I don't have to be. I know that you teach me and guide me, but only when I stop to listen to you.*
>
> *I ask you to help me recognize my complete inability to do anything of value without your help. Thank you for the freedom that this realization brings.*
>
> *I know that you can help me eat in a balanced way and that it is possible to be free of thinking about food so much if I try to use this program that I have been given. A part of me is excited about this, and another part recoils at the discipline it entails. Please put a desire in my heart to do what it takes to gain victory over my desire to eat too much. Help me focus on the fact that you will help me, one day at a time. Help me remember the harvest of righteousness and peace that awaits me.*
>
> *I surrender my will and my life to you, my God. I love you, and I trust you to do things in me that I am unable to do in my own strength. Thank you for sending Jesus to be my savior so that I don't have to be perfect. Thank you for your sufficiency, for your power at work in me, for your unconditional love.*
>
> *In Jesus' name . . .*

Read one of your Bible meditations from last week's homework assignment.

## STEPPING STONE SURVEY

We can use the Stepping Stones to help us turn away from childish behavior. Write your answers below on how each Stepping Stone can help us *step forward* toward recovery and away from the behaviors of our childhood.

Journaling _____

Honesty _____

Confidentiality _____

Prayer _____

Reaching Out _____

Fellowship _____

Accountability _____

Scripture _____

Food Plan _____

## SPIRITUAL FOCUS

This week begins our study of Step 4: **Made a searching and fearless moral inventory of ourselves.**

### How do we do this?
- We inventory our past. (This will be covered in the next three lessons.)
- We inventory our character defects. (This will be covered in the following three lessons.)

### Why do we look back when we want to step forward?
Take notes on each of the following Bible verses during the group's discussion and how the verses relate to looking back and *stepping forward*.

*John 12:46*—Jesus said, "I have come into the world as a light, so that no one who believes in me should stay in darkness."

_____

_____

*1 John 1:9*—If we confess our sins, he is faithful and just and will forgive us our sins and purify us from all unrighteousness.

_____

_____

*Psalm 51:6*—Surely you desire truth in the inner parts. You teach me wisdom in the inmost place.

_____

_____

*Lamentations 3:40*—Let us examine our ways and test them and let us return to the Lord.

_____

_____

### How can we do a Fourth Step wrong?

_____

_____

### Childhood Inventory

Let's begin our Fourth Step by doing an inventory of our childhood:

### What were our parents like?

Our purpose is not to blame our problems on our parents, but to inventory the roots of our character defects, addictions, and vicious cycles by looking at our past. Like pulling up weeds, if we snip off only the obvious results of these ineffective behaviors without digging deeper, they may not be done away with.

Look at the charts below and on the next page to take an inventory of your parents' styles of parenting. Your group leader will tell you whether to fill it out in class or as a homework assignment.

| What type of parenting style was your parents' primary one? Place a ✓ under Mon or Dad if this was their style. | | |
| --- | --- | --- |
| Style | Mom | Dad |
| Dictator | | |
| Perfectionist | | |
| Permissive (few rules) | | |
| Over-indulgent (many gifts) | | |
| Neglectful | | |
| Rejecting | | |
| Encourager | | |

---

### What were top three attributes and defects?

| Mother's attributes | Mother's defects |
|---|---|
| 1._____ | 1._____ |
| 2._____ | 2._____ |
| 3._____ | 3._____ |

| Father's attributes | Father's defects |
|---|---|
| 1._____ | 1._____ |
| 2._____ | 2._____ |
| 3._____ | 3._____ |

---

### Aren't we dishonoring our parents to talk about this?

_____

_____

### How can we forgive our prents for their weaknesses?

The last thing most of our parents wanted was to harm us. Now that many of us are parents, we can understand what a difficult task rearing children is and can forgive them for their weaknesses. But some parents did harm us intentionally, and we can forgive them too.

### How does the following verse help us to forgive our parents?

*Genesis 50:20*—You intended to harm me, but God intended it for good to accomplish what is now being done, the saving of many lives.

_____

_____

### How does a child reason? In other words, what is a child's perspective?
Read the following Bible verse from 1 Corinthians 13:11:

"When I was a child, I talked like a child, I thought like a child, I reasoned like a child. When I became a man, I put childish ways behind me."

### What are some things that a child might say when confronted with something upsetting?
Put a checkmark by the ones that you have said in the past, either to yourself or out loud.

❑ "It's all my fault."
❑ "If I were not so bad, bad things wouldn't happen."
❑ "If I don't talk about it, it will go away."

---

- ❑ "I think I'll run away."
- ❑ "I should be able to change this person."
- ❑ "Food will fix it."

*Do we still say any of these things?*

_____

_____

---

### How did we cope with the stress caused by our parents' defects?
### Circle ones that you still use:

| | |
|---|---|
| Denial | People-pleasing |
| Overeating | Striving for perfection |
| Blaming | Rebelling |
| Giving up | Frantic activities |
| Pretending, dishonesty | Isolating |

---

*How can we give up childish ways of talking, reasoning, and coping?*
Work the steps to answer this question.

*Step 1:* _____

_____

*Step 2:* _____

_____

*Step 3:* _____

_____

*Step 4:* _____

_____

*What are some ways that our misery can become ministry?*

- Our misery becomes ministry when we help others who have experienced something similar.
- Our misery becomes ministry when we overcome obstacles placed in our childhoods. Our testimonies reflect the Lord's handiwork, and we can encourage others.
- Our misery becomes ministry when we learn to rely on the Lord, because when we rely on him, he turns our weaknesses to strengths. This inspires others to rely on him too.
- Our misery becomes ministry when we are able to empathize with others in pain and show them compassion because we know how they feel.

# PHYSICAL FOCUS

*List reasons why we may have begun to eat compulsively. Write all of the reasons mentioned.*

_____

_____

_____

_____

# PRACTICING THE PRINCIPLES
(Homework)

1. Write the story of your childhood, covering years 0–12. Include the answers to the questions below and anything else significant concerning those years. Review this session and go through old photo albums to help you remember your childhood.

   - What were your parents like? What was their parenting style? What were their top three attributes and defects?
   - How are you like them?
   - How did you cope as a child?
   - Do you still cope like you did as a child?
   - How can you use the misery of your childhood for ministry? (Skip if your childhood wasn't miserable.)

2. Discuss childhood eating: Was it compulsive? Were you fat? Were you rewarded and/or consoled with food?

3. Write a Fourth Step prayer as you reflect on the verses in No. 5 (below).

4. Bring a childhood photo to class that shows what you were really like.

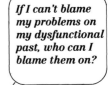

*If I can't blame my problems on my dysfunctional past, who can I blame them on?*

5. Meditate on the following verses as they relate to the Fourth Step:
   - Psalm 139:23–24
   - 2 Corinthians 9:8
   - John 8:31—32
   - Romans 13:11
   - Psalm 51:6

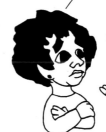
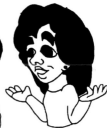

*Julie's Thoughts to Munch On*

*In Step Forward I can find the family I never had—one that will love me unconditionally, just as I am, and encourage me to become all I can be.*

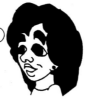

---

STEP FORWARD—*Why Should I Look Back When I Want to Step Forward?*

**Session 8:**

# Am I a 40-Year-Old Adolescent?

__GUIDING PRINCIPLE:__ *I can know who I am and can relate better to others if I inventory my adolescence.*

## APPLICATION QUESTION

*Circle a way of coping that you use that began when you were a child. What harm is this childlike behavior doing? (Try not to repeat an answer already given.)*

| | | |
|---|---|---|
| Denial | Giving Up | Rebelling |
| Overeating | Pretending | Frantic Activities |
| Blaming | People-Pleasing | Isolating |

## PRINCIPLES FROM THE WORD

Share meditations from your homework Scriptures.

Read your Fourth Step prayer.

## STEPPING STONE SURVEY

This week's Stepping Stone focus is on Fellowship. Answer this question:

*How has your group fellowship helped you physically, emotionally, or spiritually to overcome the hurts of your past?*

## SPIRITUAL FOCUS
*Healing Our Hurts*

The Fourth Step is not to fix any problems, just to inventory them. Later on in Steps 6 through 9 we will be focusing on solutions. We do want to find hope and encouragement along the way, however.

*How do each of the following Scriptures help heal the hurts of our past?*

*Romans 8:26–27*—In the same way, the Spirit helps us in our weakness. We do not know what we ought to pray for, but the Spirit himself intercedes for us with groans that words cannot express. And he who searches our hearts knows the mind of the

Spirit, because the Spirit intercedes for the saints in accordance with God's will.

_____

_____

*Isaiah 54:4*—Do not be afraid; you will not suffer shame. Do not fear disgrace; you will not be humiliated. You will forget the shame of your youth.

_____

_____

*Psalm 139:13–14*—For you created my inmost being; you knit me together in my mother's womb. I praise you because I am fearfully and wonderfully made; your works are wonderful, I know that full well.

_____

_____

*Romans 8:28*—We know that in all things God works for the good of those who love him, who have been called according to his purpose.

_____

_____

*2 Corinthians 1:3–4*—Praise be to the God and Father of our Lord Jesus Christ, the Father of compassion and the God of all comfort, who comforts us in all our troubles, so that we can comfort those in any trouble with the comfort we ourselves have received from God.

_____

_____

### Childhood Photographs

Share your childhood photos showing what you were really like.

### Adolescence

There are two tasks of adolescence: establishing our identity; and learning to be intimate. (This is not referring to sexual intimacy.)

### Establishing Our Identity: Who Are You, Really?

Individuals have to determine who they are, what they believe, what their values are, and what they think about God. When their identity is in their job, their family, or their possessions, they will crumble if these things are lost.

### Prove it!

We prove who we are by how we act in difficult circumstances. We may say one thing and act in an opposite way when the going gets rough.

### *Learning to Be Intimate: What Is Intimacy?*

Intimacy is the capacity to commit ourselves to another or to others and to continue the commitment even when to do so is difficult. It is sharing ourselves with others without wearing a mask.

### *What restricts intimacy?*
Take a minute to think of answers to this question.

_____

_____

### *Why can't you make intimacy a goal?*

_____

_____

### *How can you make it grow?*
**I can determine that I will nurture intimacy in my friendships and in my marriage by . . .**

- Taking down my mask.
- Telling the truth in love.
- Not being critical or defensive.
- Not giving unwanted advice so that others will feel safe to share with me.
- Being committed to that relationship. I can prove my commitment in many ways (such as small acts of kindness, remembering things that they are concerned about, and spending time with them).

### *Can you think of other ways to make intimacy grow?*

_____

_____

### *Me? A 40-Year-Old Adolescent?*

**You might be a 40-year-old adolescent if:**

- You don't know who you are and what your values are.
- You continue to want to only "do your own thing" and "eat, drink and be merry," not considering tomorrow.
- You don't understand real intimacy or are afraid to experience it.

### *Maturity: What's It All About?*

- Mature people know who they are by knowing *whose* they are—children of the King of Kings.

- They know their father will never leave them and don't get upset when they can't see him.

- They know that they can't always have their own way but that their Heavenly Father knows best, so they don't throw a fit when things don't go to suit them.

- They appreciate things that their Daddy does for them rather than taking everything for granted.

- They don't live in magical thinking and fantasies.

- They are disciplined enough to read and study God's Word and spend time with him, learning the lessons he wants to teach them, without daydreaming or trying to play hooky.

- When they make a mistake, they are able to face it and learn from it, rather than blaming it on someone else or lying about it.

- They are able to defer instant gratification and don't scream if they have to wait for food. They even goes hungry sometimes without pouting or complaining.

- They are able to recognize the truth, and they base their thoughts and actions on it.

- They set goals, they make plans, they accept challenges, they persevere even when it's difficult.

## PHYSICAL FOCUS

*What may have caused your overeating? Put a checkmark beside the ones that apply to you.*

- ❏ A bad habit taught by parents or peers.
- ❏ To reexperience the nurturing you felt when fed by your mother.
- ❏ To distract yourself from difficult circumstances.
- ❏ To numb your pain and comfort yourself when experiencing negative feelings.
- ❏ To create the (false) intimacy that people share when they eat together.
- ❏ To please people. (This is especially true with parents who demand that you clean your plate and eat food whether hungry or not.)
- ❏ To rebel against parents who didn't want you to eat too much.
- ❏ Associating fun and food. (The only thing you ever did that was fun was to eat.)
- ❏ Associating reward and food. (Every time you did something good, you were rewarded with food.)
- ❏ To punish yourself, subconsciously knowing that extra pounds would bring the humiliation that you "deserved."
- ❏ To put on an "overcoat of fat" to protect yourself from intimacy. (This is especially seen when someone has been molested as a child.)
- ❏ Possible genetic tendency to be a compulsive overeater.

# PRACTICING THE PRINCIPLES

(Homework)

1. Continue writing the story of your childhood up to age 21. If you haven't started, it's not too late. Get busy!

2. How did each of the following help to establish your identity during adolescence?

   - Peer influence.
   - What others thought about you.
   - Your achievements, grades, awards (or lack of).
   - Your possessions, clothes.
   - Your abilities (either scholastic or athletic).
   - Parents.

3. During adolescence who influenced you the most in a positive way? In a negative way?

4. How would you characterize yourself as a teenager? Choose three words.

5. Do you feel that you are still an adolescent? Why?

6. Review the "Physical Focus" section on the causes of overeating. Pray about each one and write about all of the reasons that may affect you.

7. Meditate on the following verses as they relate to the Fourth Step:

   - 1 Corinthians 13:11
   - Ephesians 4:14–15
   - James 1:2–6
   - Hebrews 5:13–14
   - Colossians 4:12b

**Julie's Thoughts to Munch On**

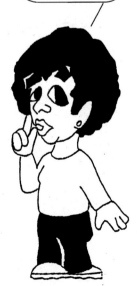

*I'm not going to tell anybody about the "real me"!*

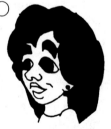

*If I keep doing the same old things, I'll keep having the same old problems.*

**Session 9:**

# What Was I Really Like?

**GUIDING PRINCIPLE:** *I can see where I got off track if I inventory my adulthood.*

## APPLICATION QUESTION

*Who influenced you the most during your adolescence? How has this affected your life?*

## PRINCIPLES FROM THE WORD

*What is the Fourth Step?*

Made a _____ and _____ moral inventory

of _____.

Review last week's homework verses from a Fourth Step perspective: As one of the following Bible verses is read, listen for the characteristics of maturity found in each verse.

*1 Corinthians 13:11*
  1. Maturity is talking as an adult.
  2. Maturity is thinking as an adult.
  3. Maturity is reasoning as an adult.

*Ephesians 3:14–16*
  4. Maturity is not forever changing one's mind.
  5. Maturity is telling the truth in love.
  6. Maturity is growing more like Jesus.

*James 1:2–6*
  7. Maturity is having faith even during trials.
  8. Maturity is showing perseverance even when times are hard.

*Hebrews 5:13–14*

9. Maturity is understanding what real righteousness is.

10. Maturity is being able to discern good from evil.

*Colossians 4:12b*

11. Maturity is standing firm in the will of God.

12. Maturity is being assured of the truth even when not apparent.

***Be prepared to share one of your meditations from last week's homework.***

***Did you bring in a childhood photo? Don't forget to show it to the rest of the group.***

## STEPPING STONE SURVEY

This week's Stepping Stone survey is covered in the Physical Focus section.

## SPIRITUAL FOCUS

This week we will take a close look at Psalm 107. Then we will use it as a medical analogy, discussing how each passage of the Scripture talks about four conditions that we deal with today in our own lives: confusion, depression, rebellion, and fear. Within each passage are found the symptoms of each condition, as well as the treatment for that condition; the results when we use that treatment; and what our response to God should be. Listen as Psalm 107 is read aloud:

Give thanks to the Lord, for he is good; his love endures forever. Let the redeemed of the Lord say this—those he redeemed from the hand of the foe, those he gathered from the lands, from east and west, from north and south. (verses 1-3)

: 4 **Some wandered in desert wastelands**, finding no way to a city where they could settle.

: 5 They were hungry and thirsty and their lives ebbed away.

: 6 Then they cried out to the Lord in their trouble and he delivered them from their distress.

: 7 He led them by a straight way to a city where they could settle.

: 8 Let them give thanks to the Lord for his unfailing love and his wonderful deeds for men,

: 9 for he satisfies the thirsty and fills the hungry with good things.

: 10 **Some sat in darkness and the deepest gloom**, prisoners suffering in iron chains,

: 11 for they had rebelled against the words of God and despised the counsel of the Most High.

: 12 So he subjected them to bitter labor; they stumbled, and there was no one to help.

: 13 Then they cried to the Lord in their trouble, and he saved them from their distress.

: 14 He brought them out of darkness and the deepest gloom and broke away their chains.

: 15 Let them give thanks to the Lord for his unfailing love and his wonderful deeds for men,

: 16 for he breaks down gates of bronze and cuts through bars of iron.

: 17 **Some became fools through their rebellious ways** and suffered affliction because of their iniquities.

: 18 They loathed all food and drew near the gates of death.

: 19 Then they cried to the Lord in their trouble, and he saved them from their distress.

: 20 He sent forth his word and healed them; he rescued them from the grave.

: 21 Let them give thanks to the Lord for his unfailing love and his wonderful deeds for men.

: 22 Let them sacrifice thank offerings and tell of his works with songs of joy.

| **Confusion** (verses 4-9) | **Depression** (verses 10-16) | **Rebellion** (verses 17-22) | **Fear** (verses 23-31) |
|---|---|---|---|
| Symptoms | Symptoms | Symptoms | Symptoms |
| 1. _____ | _____ | _____ | _____ |
| 2. _____ | _____ | _____ | _____ |
| 3. _____ | _____ | _____ | _____ |
| 4. _____ | _____ | _____ | _____ |

Treatment (verses 6, 13, 19, and 28): _____

_____

| Results | Results | Results | Results |
|---|---|---|---|
| 1. _____ | _____ | _____ | _____ |
| 2. _____ | _____ | _____ | _____ |
| 3. _____ | _____ | _____ | _____ |

Our Response (verses 8, 15, 21, and 31):_____

_____

: 23 **Others went out on the sea in ships**; they were merchants on the mighty waters. : 24 They saw the works of the Lord, his wonderful deeds in the deep.

: 25 For he spoke and stirred up a tempest that lifted high the waves.

: 26 They mounted up to the heavens and went down to the depths; in their peril their courage melted away.

: 27 They reeled and staggered like drunken men; they were at their wits' end.

: 28 Then they cried out to the Lord in their trouble, and he brought them out of their distress.

: 29 He stilled the storm to a whisper; the waves of the sea were hushed.

: 30 They were glad when it grew calm, and he guided them to their desired haven.

: 31 Let them give thanks to the Lord for his unfailing love and his wonderful deeds for men.

*Fill out the chart on the previous page during the group discussion on the Scripture.*

## PHYSICAL FOCUS

**Are you having any problems with your food plan? The list below is made up of common trouble spots we hit when trying to stay on program.**

*Can you think of how you would use a Stepping Stone to help you solve each problem?*
Try not to use the same Stepping Stones over and over. Discuss possible solutions and take notes under each problem.

**I rarely plan when or what I'm going to eat.**

_____

_____

**I eat too much at mealtime.**

_____

_____

**I snack between meals.**

_____

_____

**I sample while I cook.**

_____

_____

**I eat out often.**

_____

_____

**I don't know what gets into me, but I can't stop eating.**

_____

_____

## PRACTICING THE PRINCIPLES
(Homework)

1. It's not too late to begin writing your Fourth Step. Start writing your autobiography now.

2. While continuing to meditate on Psalm 107, write on your past, from age 21 to the time that you started your program of recovery. (We will discuss the present starting next week.) Choose one of the four categories with which you have had the most problems and answer the questions that refer to that category. If you have time, answer all the questions.

### Confusion
1. During what time(s) did you wander in a desert wasteland? (verse 4)
2. Were you eating compulsively during that time? Describe. (verse 5)
3. How did you feel that you were wasting your life? (verse 5) Did you call out to the Lord for help? (verse 6)
4. What was the "City" like where God led you to settle? Do you feel like you're still wandering? (verse 7)
5. Did you know then what God had promised? Have you claimed that promise for your life now? (verse 9)

### Depression
1. When have you felt like you were in prison? What were your chains? (verse 10)
2. Had you rebelled against God at those times? How? (verse 11)
3. How do you feel that God disciplined you? Did you resent him for it? (verse 11)
4. Did you feel that there was no one who would help you when you stumbled? Who let you down? Did you call out to God then? (verses 12-13)
5. How did he break away your chains and cut down the gates and bars of your prison? (verses 14-16)

### Rebellion
1. Have you ever rebelled against God? What were the circumstances? (verse 17)
2. What happened as a result? (verse 17)
3. Have you ever felt you were drawing near the gates of death as a result of your eating disorder or because of your rebellion? Explain. (verse 18)
4. Did you cry out to God when you were rebelling? (verse 19)
5. Has there been a time when God directly rescued you? How? (verse 20)

### Fear

1. What have been the circumstances surrounding the storms in your life? (verses 23-26)

2. Did your courage melt away? How did you feel? (verse 26)

3. During the storm, when have you been at your wit's end? (verse 27)

4. Did you cry out to the Lord? How? (verse 28)

5. How did he bring you out of your distress, still the storm, and guide you to your desired haven? (verses 29-30)

3. Meditate on the following Scriptures as they pertain to our Fourth Step:

- Psalm 107:6, 13, 19, 28
- Psalm 107:8, 15, 21, 31
- Psalm 107:35–37
- Psalm 91:9–16
- Psalm 23

*Julie's Thoughts to Munch On*

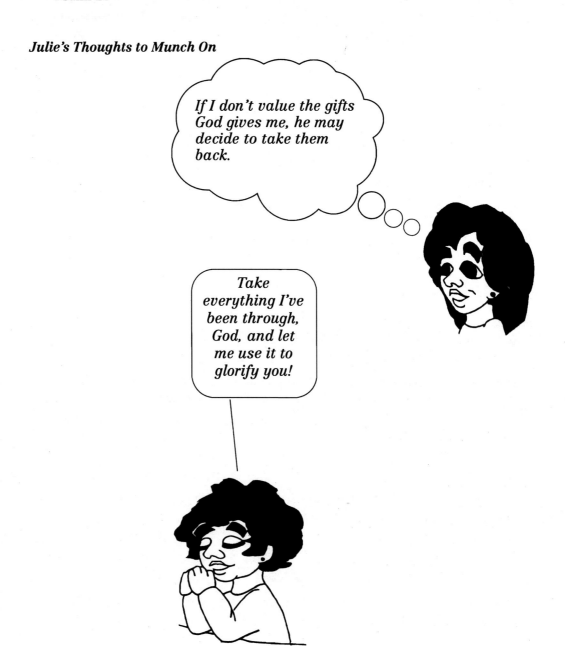

*If I don't value the gifts God gives me, he may decide to take them back.*

*Take everything I've been through, God, and let me use it to glorify you!*

**Session 10:**

# Am I Guilty As Charged?

*I can lighten my load if I inventory my guilt.*

## APPLICATION QUESTION

*Which one of the four conditions affected your life the most from age 21 until you began your program of recovery? What happened when you called out to the Lord in your trouble?*

- Confusion
- Depression
- Rebellion
- Fear

## PRINCIPLES FROM THE WORD

Discuss the homework Bible verses from a Fourth Step perspective.

## STEPPING STONE SURVEY

This week's Stepping Stone focus is on Prayer.

*How can we be encouraged to pray more?*

Following are three guidelines for prayer. Match them with instructions on why those guidelines are important by putting the letter in the space beside the guideline it goes with.

_____ Remember who God is and who we are.

_____ Praise him for the opportunity he gives us to pray.

_____ Remember answers to prayer we have experienced.

A. We have such a tendency to forget the 99 answers to prayer and remember the one we are still waiting for. It is important to record our prayers so that we can recall each answer. This not only reminds us to praise God for answering our prayers, but it also reminds us that prayer does change things.

B. So often we pray out of obligation and take for granted the fact that God is available to us any time day or night. We may doubt that our prayers are heard or that they make a difference. We may even have a "let's get this over with" attitude toward prayer. How this must hurt God!

C. God is the King of Kings and Lord of Lords, the creator of the universe, and he has chosen us to be his children. He wants us to share our thoughts and desires with him as much as we want our own children to tell us what they are thinking. Just as important, he wants us to hear his instructions, his encouragement, and his correction just as we want our children to listen to our words.

*What are some ways that we can establish good prayer habits?*

_____

_____

_____

## SPIRITUAL FOCUS

Today we will begin to inventory present character defects by discussing guilt. Discuss each question.

*Is guilt always a defect of character? Why?*

_____

_____

*How can we tell false guilt from the real thing?*

If guilt is false, it's condemnation from Satan:
- It's non–specific.
- It's hopeless.
- There's no way out of the situation.

If guilt is real, it's conviction from the Holy Spirit:
- It's specific.
- It comes with hope.
- There's a way out — a plan eventually comes when we pray.

*What does this statement imply: "I know that God forgives me, but I can't forgive myself."*

_____

_____

*What happens if one has too much guilt? Circle the ones that apply to you.*

Legalism—trying to earn salvation through good works

Fear—of hell and God's rejection

Doubt God's mercy

Try to run from God

Rationalize

Make excuses

Blame others

Be ashamed of self

Rebel ("I can't please him anyway")

Be depressed (anger at self)

Don't appreciate God's amazing grace

Be a poor testimony

## *What happens if one has too little guilt?*

Disobedience

Unconfessed sin

Hardness toward God

Numbness to the Holy Spirit

God does not hear our prayers

God turns his face from us when we sin

Poor testimony

No service to others; not useful to God

Bad influence on others

God disciplines us

Limited reward in heaven

We miss out on the richness of God's blessings

## *How do I draw the line between the two extremes?*

- The Bible
- The Holy Spirit

## *What is sin?*

_____

_____

## *What is grace? (Consider both verses before you answer.)*

*Ephesians 2:8*—For it is by grace you have been saved, through faith—and this not from yourselves it is the gift of God— not by works, so that no one can boast.

*2 Corinthians 9:8*—God is able to make all grace abound to you, so that in all things at all times, having all that you need, you will abound in every good work.

_____

_____

*What is righteousness?*

_____

_____

### Name two types of righteousness.

- **Justification:** God sees us just as though we have never sinned as soon as we confess Christ as our savior.

  *Romans 3:22–24a* —This righteousness from God comes through faith in Jesus Christ to all who believe. There is no difference, for all have sinned and fall short of the glory of God and are justified freely by his grace.

- **Sanctification:** the process of becoming more like Christ. This is a transformation that continues throughout our lifetime—it happens when we are abiding in the Lord and relying on his grace to give us the willingness and ability to be obedient to his Word.

  *1 Thessalonians 4:1a, 3a* —Finally, brothers, we instructed you how to live in order to please God. . . . It is God's will that you should be sanctified . . .

### What attitude should I have concerning righteousness?

- A desire to *step forward,* a willingness to work at it, and a teachable spirit.

  *Philippians 3:12  (The Living Bible)*—I don't mean to say I am perfect. I haven't learned all I should even yet, but I keep working toward that day when I will finally be all that Christ saved me for and wants me to be.

- A desire not to sin, but recognizing our need for a savior. An appreciation of Jesus' perfect atonement for us on the cross.

  *1 John 2:1–2a* —My dear children, I write this to you so that you will not sin. But if anybody does sin, we have one who speaks to the Father in our defense—Jesus Christ, the Righteous One. He is the atoning sacrifice for our sins . . .

### What does this all have to do with stepping forward?

I am saved by Jesus alone, not by my good deeds or my nice personality. But because I trust in his sacrifice on the cross, I want to do what God wants me to do. As I focus on God and his Word and rely on the Holy Spirit for the desire and the ability to obey him, I slowly become more like Jesus. Sometimes I fail and slip back into my old ways and, when I do, I confess this to God, and he forgives me. When I trust in Jesus' atonement for my sins, I am able to live in his grace and experience the freedom to be all that God calls me to be.

### How should I confess my sins?

Read and compare the information in the two boxes below, "A Modern Sinner Confesses" and "How a Christian Confesses."

## "A Modern Sinner Confesses"
### (or "How Not to Confess Sin")

:1    Forgive me, God, because I was reared in a dysfunctional family and can't help myself.
:2    And I haven't hurt anyone else.
:3    Thank you God, that you are not judgmental and that you accept everyone no matter what we do.
:4    You created my desires and so it is good to express them.
:5    I am human and have no choice but to be myself.
:6    Surely you desire that I am true to my inner self.
:7    If something feels good, it is good.
:8    Make me happy, God. Make me feel good about myself.
:9    I know that all I have to do is say, "I'm sorry," and anything I continue to do is okay.
:10   Create in me a happy heart, O God. I deserve it because I am basically a good person.
:11   Don't take my good life away from me.
:12   Restore to me the happiness that I had before and grant me my desires.
:16   I know that you appreciate the sacrifice I make two Sundays a month when I go to church and the money that I have given.
:17   Thank you that you don't despise anyone and that your forgiveness is universal.

## How a Christian Confesses
### (Psalm 51)

:1    Have mercy on me, O god, according to your unfailing love; according to your great compassion blot out my transgressions.

:2    Wash away all my iniquity and cleanse me from my sin.

:3    For I know my transgressions, and my sin is always before me.

:4    Against you, you only, have I sinned and done what is evil in your sight, so that you are proved right  when you speak and justified when you judge.

:5    Surely I was sinful at birth, sinful from the time my mother conceived me.

:6    Surely you desire truth in the inner parts; you teach me wisdom in the inmost place.

:7    Cleanse me with hyssop, and I will be clean; wash me, and I will be whiter than snow.

:8    Let me hear with joy and gladness, let the bones you have crushed rejoice.

:9    Hide your face from my sins and blot out my iniquity.

:10   Create in me a pure heart, O God, and renew a right spirit within me.

:11   Do not cast me from your presence or take your Holy Spirit from me.

:12   Restore to me the joy of your salvation and grant me a willing spirit to sustain me.

:16   You do not delight in sacrifice, or I would bring it; you do not take pleasure in burnt offerings.

:17   The sacrifices of God are a broken spirit; a broken and contrite heart, O God, you will not despise.

*What are the differences between how a modern sinner confesses and how a Christian confesses? In each pair of statements, put a plus beside the one that is how a Christian confesses. Put a minus beside the one that is how a modern sinner confesses.*

\_\_\_\_ Blames others and makes excuses.

\_\_\_\_ Accepts responsibility for his or her sin.


\_\_\_\_ Recognizes any harm and pleads for mercy.

\_\_\_\_ Denies any harm he or she has done.


\_\_\_\_ Knows that God is loving and that he also judges him or her.

\_\_\_\_ Knows that God is loving and assumes that means he does not judge.


\_\_\_\_ Thinks the law is old-fashioned and restricting.

\_\_\_\_ Knows that God's law never changes and is for his or her good.


\_\_\_\_ Praises God for his forgiveness and knows that it is received only through God's grace.

\_\_\_\_ Tries to earn forgiveness.


## PHYSICAL FOCUS

*Answer the questions in "How Am I Doing?" on p. 61.*


## PRACTICING THE PRINCIPLES
(Homework)

1. Write a meditation on the following:

   "God loves me just the way I am, but he loves me too much to leave me the way I am."

2. Continue your Fourth Step inventory:

   • List the things that you have felt guilty over this week. Note next to each one if you feel that this was condemnation from the accuser or conviction from the Holy Spirit. Praise God for his forgiveness in Christ.

   • List any sins that you have not been able to forgive yourself for. As you meditate on 1 John 1:9, confess them and stand firm against the accuser when he tries to convince you that you are not forgiven.

   • List any sins that you continue in and are unwilling to give up. Write a prayer confessing this to God and asking him to give you the willingness you need.

   • List any sins that you continue to repent of but frequently fall back into. Write a prayer asking God for the ability to turn from these sins in his strength.

3. Memorize 1 John 1:9.

4. Meditate on the following in light of God's forgiveness.

- Psalm 51:16–17
- 1 John 1:9
- Ephesians 2:8–9
- Colossians 1:21–23*a*
- Matthew 9:12–13

*Julie's Thoughts to Munch On*

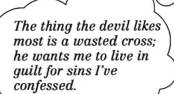

*The thing the devil likes most is a wasted cross; he wants me to live in guilt for sins I've confessed.*

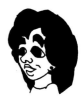

# How Am I Doing?
Choose the best answer for each question.

**How is my eating?**
1. I usually eat according to my food plan and the cravings are almost all gone.
2. I never binge anymore, but I still have occasional slips.
3. I try, but I can't seem to stop binging occasionally.
4. I'm not even trying to eat less.

**How is my weight?**
1. I am consistently losing weight or am at my goal weight.
2. I lose only a pound or so a month.
3. I am maintaining my weight, but I still need to lose.
4. I am gaining weight.

**How is my exercise?**
1. I exercise four or five times a week for more than 20 minutes.
2. I exercise only two or three times a week for more than 20 minutes.
3. I want to, but I don't have a consistent exercise program. I am exercising occasionally though.
4. I'm not trying to exercise at this time.

**How is my program?**
1. I'm trying to use most of the Stepping Stones and am taking the steps by taking careful notes in class; doing the assignments; and practicing the principles I am learning.
2. I'm having quiet times almost every day, and I call a coach or accountability partner at least two times a week.
3. I come to the meetings every week and do some of the assignments.
4. I am auditing Step Forward (not doing the assignments) and come to the meetings when something else doesn't come up.

**What am I willing to do to?**
1. I am willing to commit to using at least six Stepping Stones every day.
2. I am willing to use two of the Stepping Stones every day.
3. I am willing to try to come to meetings more consistently.
4. I am willing to pray for willingness to put my recovery before other things that keep me too busy to do what I know I need to do.

## Score your test by adding the number next to each answer given.
5–7     Great! Keep up the good work!
8–10    You're working program. With just a little more effort, you'll see more weight loss.
11–13   Call your group leader or your coach and get help in setting new goals. Don't be discouraged!
14–20   Keep coming back. Don't give up. If you want to get help, don't hesitate to call your group leader. If you want to audit, it's okay. Your time will come. Keep praying for willingness.

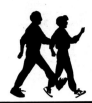

**Session 11:**

# I'm Not Resentful, Just Hurt!

---

**GUIDING PRINCIPLE:** *I can forgive if I inventory my resentments.*

## APPLICATION QUESTION

*"God loves me just the way I am, but he loves me too much to leave me the way I am." What one thing (other than your overeating) do you think that God wants to change in you most? Share your meditation on this statement if you wrote one.*

## PRINCIPLES FROM THE WORD

Discuss the Bible verses from last week's homework assignment. Share your meditation on one of the verses.

## STEPPING STONE SURVEY

This week's Stepping Stone focus is on Journaling. One way we journal is by using our Victory List. Let's review from Unit 1 how we use our Victory List:

We list five short-term goals that we want to accomplish and put an X under each day that we achieve that goal. Our Victory List reminds us to pray for willingness and ability to do each item, and it encourages us to *step forward* in our program and to be accountable.

*Other Ways to Use the Victory List*

• Try using the monthly Victory List found in the back of your workbook.

• Increase your number of short-term goals to 10 or 12 if you have been using your Victory List. If you have not been using your Victory List, begin with only five goals. If a goal is new or particularly difficult, give yourself double or triple points if you accomplish it. You may do this by putting an X in the block under that day in a different color to remind you that it is worth more. This gives you a double incentive.

• Celebrate your victories. If you make a high percentage of your goals or *step forward* in a particularly difficult area, reward yourself (of course, not with food!). Be creative in your rewards. Ask yourself what you want to have (that's affordable) or what you would like to do (that's permissible) to reward yourself when you achieve your goal.

---

- Even small incentives help. My accountability partner and I give each other stickers when we do exceptionally well that week. Another thing that will encourage you is to tell your group about a goal you are trying to reach and then tell them when you reach it.
- Be careful when using your Victory List that you don't get perfectionistic. Don't attempt to get 100 percent every time. This encourages the all-or-nothing mentality. Then you may find yourself saying, "If I didn't do it perfectly, I may as well do it terribly!" Don't berate yourself if you don't achieve your goals or make your goals so difficult that you'll never be able to do them. Make your goals achievable and then plan to *step forward* from there.

## SPIRITUAL FOCUS

### Resentment

**Resentment is refusal to let go of anger over some past harm.**

*What are some usual causes of resentment?*

_____

_____

*What are some ways that we express resentment?*

_____

_____

### Forgiveness

God has a goal for our resentments: It's call forgiveness. Forgiveness is defined as "giving up your perceived right to punish the one who has offended you, canceling a debt owed to you." Forgiveness is a choice, not a feeling.

What does Satan come to tell us about forgiveness? He comes to tell us that we should not forgive, cannot forgive, or have not forgiven a person.

### What does the Bible say about forgiveness?

**The Results of Unforgiveness:** Read the following verses. Discuss and list under each one what happens in our lives when we refuse to forgive others.

- *Matthew 18:21–35:* Read this passage.

   **Results of unforgiveness:**

_____

_____

_____

- *Hebrews 12:1*—Let us throw off everything that hinders and the sin that so easily entangles.

    **Results of unforgiveness:**

    _____

    _____

- *Hebrews 12:15*—See to it that no one misses the grace of God and that no bitter root grows up to cause trouble and defile many.

    **Results of unforgiveness:**

    _____

    _____

- *Psalm 66:18*—If I cherish sin in my heart, God won't hear my prayers.

    **Results of unforgiveness:**

    _____

    _____

- *Ephesians 4:26–27*—In your anger do not sin: do not let the sun go down while you are still angry and do not give the devil a foothold.

    **Results of unforgiveness:**

    _____

    _____

**The Rewards of Forgiveness:**
Read the verses, discuss them, and list under each one the rewards we experience when we forgive others.

- *Luke 6:32–35*—If you love those who love you, what credit is that to you? Even "sinners" love those who love them . . . Love your enemies, do good to them, and lend to them without expecting to get anything back. Then your reward will be great and you will be sons of the Most High. . . .

    **Rewards of forgiveness:**

    _____

    _____

- *Luke 6:37–38*—Do not judge and you will not be judged. Do not condemn and you will not be condemned. Forgive and you will be forgiven. Give and it will be given to you, a good measure, pressed down, shaken together, running over will be poured into your lap. For with the measure you use, it will be measured to you.

**Rewards of forgiveness:**

_____

_____

## Instructions on How to Forgive

Read the verses, discuss them, and list under each one specific instructions concerning how to forgive.

- *Mark 11:23–25*—I tell you the truth, if anyone says to this mountain, "Go throw yourself into the sea," and does not doubt in his heart but believes that what he says will happen, it will be done for him. Therefore I tell you, whatever you ask for in prayer, believe that you have received it, and it will be yours. And when you stand praying, if you hold anything against anyone, forgive him, so that your Father in heaven may forgive you your sins.

**Instructions on how to forgive:**

_____

_____

*Why do you think Jesus used the mountain in the sea analogy before he talked about forgiving?*

_____

_____

*Does the last sentence in this passage mean that we won't go to heaven if we live in resentment?*

_____

_____

- *Luke 6:41–2*—Why do you look at the speck of sawdust in your brother's eye and pay no attention to the plank in your own eye? . . . You hypocrite, first take the plank out of your own eye and then you will see clearly to remove the speck from your brother's eye.

**Instructions on how to forgive:**

_____

_____

*Do you ever criticize someone for something that you do yourself? Why?*

_____

- *Matthew 18:21–22*—Then Peter came to Jesus and asked, "Lord, how many times shall I forgive my brother when he sins against me? Up to seven times?" Jesus answered, "I tell you, not seven times, but seventy-seven times."

**Instructions on how to forgive:**

_____

_____

- *Luke 17:3a*—If your brother sins rebuke him . . .

**Instructions on how to forgive:**

_____

_____

*Which of our Stepping Stones is being referred to here? What happens if we don't use this? How can we do this wrong?*

_____

_____

- *Hebrews 12:2a*—Let us fix our eyes on Jesus, the author and perfecter of our faith . . .

**Instructions on how to forgive:**

_____

_____

- **Romans 12:20–21**—If your enemy is hungry, feed him; if he is thirsty, give him something to drink. In doing this, you will heap burning coals on his head.

**Instructions on how to forgive:**

_____

_____

_____

*How can we do this with the wrong motivation?*

_____

_____

_____

Keeping this verse in mind, practice the "nice game" (see below for how it's played). This will improve any relationship!

---

## The Nice Game

- Do one nice thing a day for your husband, mother, boss, or whomever you are struggling to forgive.
- If you complain that they didn't notice or reciprocate, you don't "get credit"!
- You must do different things every day. This will help you to be constantly thinking about what they need so that you can do your "nice thing."
  ** *The same "nice things" can be repeated the following week.*

---

*Remember this life-changing reminder:*

*"I cannot change anyone else. I can only change myself but, often when I change, the other person does too!"*

*Tackle Resentment by Working the Steps*

1. I admit that I am I powerless over my resentments and that my life can become unmanageable because of them.
2. I am coming to believe that God through Jesus Christ can help me to forgive.
3. I am making a decision to turn these resentments over to God by working my program (doing the Anger Action Plan, praying, journaling, and so forth).
4. I am making a list of all of my resentments.
5. I am sharing this with God and another.

# PHYSICAL FOCUS

*Share steps forward that you have taken in the physical part of your program.*

# PRACTICING THE PRINCIPLES
(Homework)

1. Review the results of unforgiveness, the rewards of forgiveness, and instruction on how to forgive.

2. If you are overwhelmed with resentment, especially toward one particular person, go through the Anger Action Plan (see Unit 1, Session 6) concerning this person while praying that God will enable you to forgive. Skip No. 3.

3. If you are not overwhelmed at present, make a Grudge List. Do not dig up old resentments that you have already worked through. Do this only after praying that God will protect you from Satan, who wants you to get overwhelmed in your resentments. Make a list of people toward whom you feel resentful. Briefly state why you are angry and how you feel about yourself as a result of their actions. Work through the Anger Action Plan with as many of them as you can.

4. Write a prayer that God will forgive you of the sin of resentment and give you the grace to enable you to forgive each person on your list.

5. Choose five verses from this lesson and write a meditation on them.

***Julie's Thoughts to Munch On***

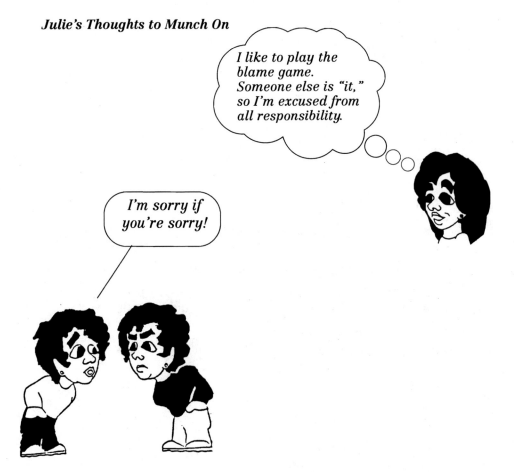

*STEP FORWARD—I'm Not Resentful, Just Hurt!*

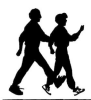

**Session 12:**

# Me . . . Lustful?

**GUIDING PRINCIPLE:** *I can learn how to control my appetites if I inventory my lust.*

## APPLICATION QUESTION

*With whom do you have the greatest problem of resentment? Name one way that these resentments have harmed you.*

## PRINCIPLES FROM THE WORD

Share your Bible meditations from your homework and any *steps forward* toward forgiveness that you have made as a result of working program.

## STEPPING STONE SURVEY

The goal of the Step Forward program is to help each member do the following every day:

• Recognize and admit my weaknesses, mistakes, and sins.
• Recognize the negative consequences of these behaviors.
• Draw close to God and cooperate with him.
• Experience God's transforming grace.

*How has a Stepping Stone helped you to step forward toward one of these objectives?*

(Do not discuss a Stepping Stone already mentioned until all of them have been discussed.)

## SPIRITUAL FOCUS

We will complete our Fourth Step introduction by discussing lust. Lust is defined as "an overwhelming desire for something."

*What are some things that people lust for?*

_____

_____

*What makes lust worse?*

If you tried to deal with your lust by working the steps incorrectly — with a negative twist — it would look something like this:

Step 1—I don't admit my powerlessness over lust and refuse to recognize how it is affecting my life.

Step 2—I don't think God can help me turn from lust.

Step 3—I have made a decision to either give up completely or to try harder with willpower to refrain from my lust.

Step 4—I won't think about what I am doing, so I won't have to deal with my lust.

Step 5—I won't share anything about my lust with anyone and will just pretend that God isn't looking when I choose to indulge in it.

**Read the following Scripture from Deuteronomy 8:2–3:**

"Remember how the Lord your God led you all the way in the desert these 40 years to humble you and to test you in order to know what was in your heart, whether or not you would keep his commands. He humbled you, causing you to hunger then feeding you with manna, to teach you that man does not live on bread alone but on every word that comes from the mouth of the Lord."

*Based on that Scripture, why does God allow us to be tempted?*

_____

_____

*Before God can help us to stand firm against lust, which truths must be accepted?*

Look at the two verses below. Look for the truth found in each verse that must be accepted in order to receive the help that the Lord has for us in standing firm against our lust for food.

*John 10:10*—I have come that they may have life, and have it to the full.

_____

_____

*1 John 1:9*—If we confess our sins, he is faithful and just and will forgive us our sins and purify us from all unrighteousness.

_____

_____

## How might we keep from confessing our sins?

• Blame it on others (or our busy schedule!).

• Excuse it. ("I was born with a low metabolism rate.")

• Deny it. ("I'm not really fat. I carry it well. These extra pounds are not harming me.")

• Rationalize it. ("I wouldn't want to look like those malnourished skinny people. Society puts too much emphasis on thinness.")

## If we refuse to take responsibility for our sins, what happens?

_____

_____

Look at Luke 1:37 — Nothing is impossible with God!

## What step is this?
(Circle the answer.)    1    2    3    4    5

Look at 1 Corinthians 10:13 — No temptation has seized you except what is common to man. And God is faithful; he will not let you be tempted beyond what you can bear. But when you are tempted, he will also provide a way out so that you can stand up under it.

## What does this verse say about getting past temptation?

_____

_____

## Why do we fail so often in tapping God's resources? (The answers can be found in the following verses.)

*Philippians 3:18—19*—I have often told you before and now say again even with tears, many live as enemies of the cross of Christ. Their destiny is destruction, their god is their stomach and their glory is in their shame. Their mind is on earthly things.

_____

*James 1:6*—When he asks God, he must believe and not doubt, because he who doubts is like a wave of the sea, blown and tossed by the wind. That man should not think he will receive anything from the Lord; he is a double-minded man, unstable in all he does.

_____

*Psalm 86:11*—Teach me your way, O Lord, and I will walk in your truth; give me an undivided heart that I may fear your name.

_____

*James 1:2—4*—Consider it pure joy whenever you face trials of many kinds, because you know that the testing of your faith develops perseverance. Perseverance must finish its work so that you may be mature and complete, not lacking anything.

_____

*Hebrews 11:1*—Now faith is being sure of what we hope for and certain of what we do not see.

_____

*How has our food addiction helped us to mature?*
*Is it possible to eat according to your food plan and still not feel deprived?*

_____

_____

*How does an attitude of faith affect our lust?*

1. If we have faith, we understand that God gives us commands that are for our good, and we are wise to obey him.
2. We remember that anything that God commands us to do, he enables us to do.
3. We know that when we get off track and confess it, God forgives us.
4. We will never give up on ourselves because God never gives up on us.

*What are some Step Forward sayings we've learned that encourage our faith as we work our program of recovery? Match the beginning of each statement with its ending.*

"Just for today, _____ ."

"I can't. God can. _____ ."

"Food won't _____ ."

"I don't have to be perfect . . . _____ ."

"Any weakness that makes me lean on God more _____ ."

"My food plan is not for my restriction, _____ ."

| | |
|---|---|
| . . . fix it. | . . . but for my protection. |
| . . . I'm letting him! | . . . is an asset. |
| . . . I will eat right. | . . . just *step forward*. |

## PHYSICAL FOCUS

*How much do you know about losing weight? Circle either "true" or "false" for each statement.*

As long as I continue to eat between 25 and 30 grams of fat, I will lose weight.
True or false?

Skipping meals does not affect the amount of fat that is stored by my body.
True or false?

If I gain extra pounds, no harm is done as long as I lose them. True or false?

More than 300,000 people die prematurely in the United States from conditions related to weight. True or false?

The number of overweight children is only slightly higher than it was in 1970. True or false?

## PRACTICING THE PRINCIPLES
(Homework)

1. In addition to food, in what other areas do you experience an overpowering desire?

2. Do you really believe that God can help you to eat right one day at a time? Do you think that you will reach goal weight and stay there? Why or why not?

3. Refer to the section, "Why do we fail so often in tapping God's resources?" Which of the five reasons given affects your program the most? What are you going to do about it?

4. Meditate on the following verses as they relate to lust issues:
   • Numbers 11:4–6
   • Numbers 11:18–20
   • Romans 12:1–2
   • Proverbs 23:20–21
   • 1 John 2:15–16

5. Sign up for the next section in this series so you can continue *stepping forward*!

*Julie's Thoughts to Munch On*

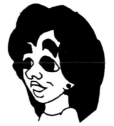

*The more I eat, the hungrier I get. I'll never be satisfied until I rely on the Spirit to fill me.*

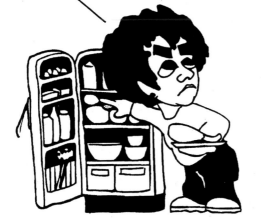

*But I thought that lust was only about sex!*

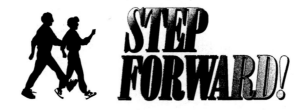

# CALORIE CONTENT

| Item | Calories |
|------|----------|
| Meat, 1 ounce, lean | 55 |
| Meat, 1 ounce, medium | 75 |
| Meat, 1 ounce, marbled | 100 |
| Bread, 1 serving | 80 |
| Fruit, 1 serving | 60 |
| Vegetable, serving | 25 |
| Milk, 8 ounces, skim | 90 |
| Milk, 8 ounces, 2 percent | 120 |
| Milk, 8 ounces, 4 percent | 150 |
| Mayonnaise, 1 tablespoon | 100 |
| Peanut butter, 1 tablespoon | 100 |
| Egg, large | 75 |
| Vegetable oil, 1 tablespoon | 120 |
| Cheese, 1 ounce | 100 (approx.) |

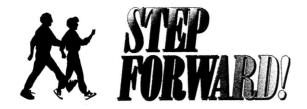

# Food Journal
## Week of _____

# One Day at a time. . .

### Day 1

| Planned: | Fat(g) | Cal | Portions |
|---|---|---|---|
| **Breakfast** | | | — Meat |
| **Lunch** | | | — Dairy / — Fruit |
| **Dinner** | | | — Veg / — Bread |
| **Snacks** | | | — Water (glasses) |
| | — | — | Totals |

| Actual: | Fat(g) | Cal | Portions |
|---|---|---|---|
| **Breakfast** | | | — Meat |
| **Lunch** | | | — Dairy / — Fruit |
| **Dinner** | | | — Veg / — Bread |
| **Snacks** | | | — Water (glasses) |
| | — | — | Totals |

**Review:**
Was my eating. . .
__ well balanced?
__ planned?
__ compulsive
__ too much  __ grazing
__ too fast  __ seconds
__ standing  __ bingeing
__ triggerfood
__ emotional
__ other
Exercise?
type _____
duration _____

### Day 2

| Planned: | Fat(g) | Cal | Portions |
|---|---|---|---|
| **Breakfast** | | | — Meat |
| **Lunch** | | | — Dairy / — Fruit |
| **Dinner** | | | — Veg / — Bread |
| **Snacks** | | | — Water (glasses) |
| | — | — | Totals |

| Actual: | Fat(g) | Cal | Portions |
|---|---|---|---|
| **Breakfast** | | | — Meat |
| **Lunch** | | | — Dairy / — Fruit |
| **Dinner** | | | — Veg / — Bread |
| **Snacks** | | | — Water (glasses) |
| | — | — | Totals |

**Review:**
Was my eating. . .
__ well balanced?
__ planned?
__ compulsive
__ too much  __ grazing
__ too fast  __ seconds
__ standing  __ bingeing
__ triggerfood
__ emotional
__ other
Exercise?
type _____
duration _____

### Day 3

| Planned: | Fat(g) | Cal | Portions |
|---|---|---|---|
| **Breakfast** | | | — Meat |
| **Lunch** | | | — Dairy / — Fruit |
| **Dinner** | | | — Veg / — Bread |
| **Snacks** | | | — Water (glasses) |
| | — | — | Totals |

| Actual: | Fat(g) | Cal | Portions |
|---|---|---|---|
| **Breakfast** | | | — Meat |
| **Lunch** | | | — Dairy / — Fruit |
| **Dinner** | | | — Veg / — Bread |
| **Snacks** | | | — Water (glasses) |
| | — | — | Totals |

**Review:**
Was my eating. . .
__ well balanced?
__ planned?
__ compulsive
__ too much  __ grazing
__ too fast  __ seconds
__ standing  __ bingeing
__ triggerfood
__ emotional
__ other
Exercise?
type _____
duration _____

**Planned:**    Fat(g)   Cal   **Portions**

Breakfast

Lunch

Dinner

Snacks

—— Meat
—— Dairy
—— Fruit
—— Veg
—— Bread
—— Water (glasses)
—— —— **Totals**

**Actual:**    Fat(g)   Cal   **Portions**

Breakfast

Lunch

Dinner

Snacks

—— Meat
—— Dairy
—— Fruit
—— Veg
—— Bread
—— Water (glasses)
—— —— **Totals**

**Review:**
Was my eating. . .
__ well balanced?
__ planned?
__ compulsive
__ too much __ grazing
__ too fast __ seconds
__ standing __ bingeing
__ triggerfood
__ emotional
__ other
Exercise?
type _____
duration _____

---

**Planned:**    Fat(g)   Cal   **Portions**

Breakfast

Lunch

Dinner

Snacks

—— Meat
—— Dairy
—— Fruit
—— Veg
—— Bread
—— Water (glasses)
—— —— **Totals**

**Actual:**    Fat(g)   Cal   **Portions**

Breakfast

Lunch

Dinner

Snacks

—— Meat
—— Dairy
—— Fruit
—— Veg
—— Bread
—— Water (glasses)
—— —— **Totals**

**Review:**
Was my eating. . .
__ well balanced?
__ planned?
__ compulsive
__ too much __ grazing
__ too fast __ seconds
__ standing __ bingeing
__ triggerfood
__ emotional
__ other
Exercise?
type _____
duration _____

---

**Planned:**    Fat(g)   Cal   **Portions**

Breakfast

Lunch

Dinner

Snacks

—— Meat
—— Dairy
—— Fruit
—— Veg
—— Bread
—— Water (glasses)
—— —— **Totals**

**Actual:**    Fat(g)   Cal   **Portions**

Breakfast

Lunch

Dinner

Snacks

—— Meat
—— Dairy
—— Fruit
—— Veg
—— Bread
—— Water (glasses)
—— —— **Totals**

**Review:**
Was my eating. . .
__ well balanced?
__ planned?
__ compulsive
__ too much __ grazing
__ too fast __ seconds
__ standing __ bingeing
__ triggerfood
__ emotional
__ other
Exercise?
type _____
duration _____

---

**Planned:**    Fat(g)   Cal   **Portions**

Breakfast

Lunch

Dinner

Snacks

—— Meat
—— Dairy
—— Fruit
—— Veg
—— Bread
—— Water (glasses)
—— —— **Totals**

**Actual:**    Fat(g)   Cal   **Portions**

Breakfast

Lunch

Dinner

Snacks

—— Meat
—— Dairy
—— Fruit
—— Veg
—— Bread
—— Water (glasses)
—— —— **Totals**

**Review:**
Was my eating. . .
__ well balanced?
__ planned?
__ compulsive
__ too much __ grazing
__ too fast __ seconds
__ standing __ bingeing
__ triggerfood
__ emotional
__ other
Exercise?
type _____
duration _____

# BATTLE PLAN

## How can we fight spiritual warfare? Read on:

1. **Pray**—*out loud or in writing.*

    **Adoration**—Look at the promises in Week 4 and thank God that they're true.

    **Confession**—Get it all out and then thank God that your sin is forgiven (1 John 1:9).

    **Thanksgiving**—Make a gratitude list of at least 20 items.

    **Supplication**—Remember Ephesians 6 "Pray, pray, pray! When you've finished, pray some more!"
    Ask God to protect you from Satan and to help you to put on God's full armor!

2. **Call your accountability partner or someone else who knows the Word.** Do not focus on "Why me?", but on "What would you have me learn?" (In other words, get off of your pity pot and get to work!) Pray together, even if only on the phone.

3. **Remember that this will pass (James 4:7).** Think of a battle, when the bombs are dropping, and so forth. Thank God that peace will come, but in the meantime there are important things that you must do to fight victoriously.

4. **Go where you can be alone.** Pray for God's wisdom (Psalm 32:8) and protection from Satan as he tries to distract you, confuse you, and make you feel overwhelmed. Take the phone off the hook. Get out your notebook, Bible, and some notebook paper.

5. **Make a "frowny face" like the one below.** Make an arrow for each of your problems and anything that is bothering you.

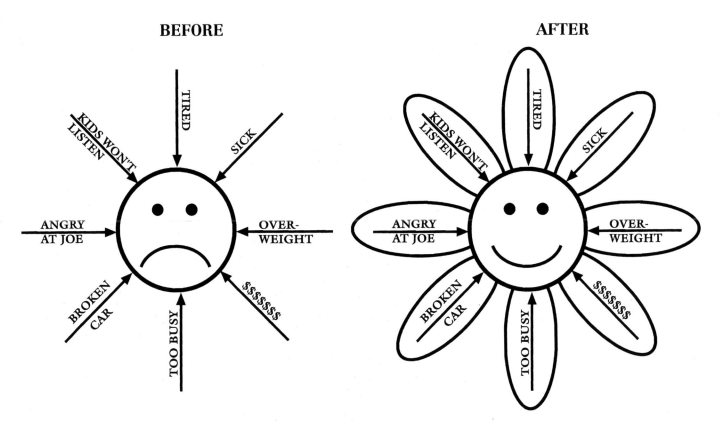

**BEFORE**　　　　　　　　　　　　**AFTER**

6. Go back to your arrow picture. **Draw "shields" around each problem that you have no control over and place those problems on your Miracle List to pray about daily.** As you are drawing the shields, thank God that he is able and willing to take care of these things for you. Ask him to help you to leave these problems in his care.

7. **Write Action Plans concerning each of the other problems.** (You may wish to do this with your accountability partner's help.) Remember the parts of an action plan:

   a. **Problem** *(Must be your problem, not someone else's—for example, not "My husband screams at me," but "I'm angry that my husband screams at me.")*

   b. **Goal** *(Must be realistic—for example, not "I won't get angry," but "I will begin the process of forgiving my husband with the Lord's help.")*

   c. **Actions** *(Must be achievable and specific—for example, not "I'll never say negative things to my husband," but "When my husband screams at me, I will pray before I respond.")*

8. **Draw a shield around each problem over which you have written an Action Plan.** Then pray that God will help you to do the things that you can with his help to resolve these problems.

9. **Place some of the specific actions from your Action Plans on your Victory List** to remind yourself of your new goals. Pray over these daily. (Just pick a few. You don't have to do this perfectly.)

10. **Now ask yourself,** *"What did I do that might have made me more vulnerable to attack?"* (Look at the lesson in Session 5 to remind you.) This is important so that you won't continue to repeat the same mistakes.

11. **Review** the lessons in Sessions 5 and 6.

12. **Pray again that God will protect you and guide you as you go about your day.** After you have shared your feelings with God and your accountability partner, don't continue to speak negatively about your problems. Each time they come back to your mind, recognize the author of those negative feelings and stand firm against him. (Take those thoughts captive!)

13. **Repeat your memory verses,** listen to praise songs, and thank God often for what he's doing in your life.

14. **Be gentle with yourself for the next few days.** Do not take on any extra obligations. Don't put yourself in a position where you will be more tempted with food. Get plenty of rest. Take extra time just to be still with the Lord. Review your verses daily. Write them where you will see them often. Don't allow the accuser to tell you that you are too busy for a quiet time.

15. If you continue to feel overwhelmed, **talk to your pastor or a Christian counselor.**

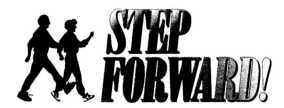

# STEP FORWARD STUCK SHEET

*Use this sheet when you can't seem to eat consistently according to your food plan. If you are willing to use the stuck sheet, you are encouraged to agree to do one short assignment every day for seven days and to talk to your coach or group leader daily during this time to read what you've written to them.*

**Day One:** Write the ways that compulsive overeating is harming you—physically, spiritually, and emotionally. Write a short prayer asking God to help you to have the willingness to stop harming yourself.

**Day Two:** What reasons do you use to give yourself permission to overeat? List ways to overcome each of these excuses. Write a short prayer asking God to help you ONE DAY AT A TIME to choose to turn from making excuses.

**Day Three:** Do you remember the question that Jesus asked the paralytic: "Do you want to be healed?" Write an honest answer to this question. List what overeating (or being overweight) is doing to "help" you. Write a prayer expressing the desire to rely on God, and not food, to get you through the hard times.

**Day Four:** See if you can list each of the Stepping Stones from memory. How are you presently using each one? Write a prayer for willingness to step forward in using them.

**Day Five:** Looking at yesterday's assignment, list how you want to use each of the Stepping Stones to work a better program. Don't make your goals too hard. Write a prayer to read daily in which you ask God to help you JUST FOR TODAY to do those things.

**Day Six:** Make a Victory List in which you list the new goals you established yesterday. Watch that you don't get legalistic about it (basing your acceptance by God on what you are or are not doing). Write a prayer thanking God for his unconditional love for you.

**Day Seven:** List the steps forward that you have taken since starting the program. Write a prayer thanking God for what he has done and is going to do in your life as you work program ONE DAY AT A TIME.

Step Forward

# Victory List

Month of ——————

*One day at a time . . . .*

**Goals:**

| | 1 | 2 | 3 | 4 | 5 | 6 | 7 | 8 | 9 | 10 | 11 | 12 | 13 | 14 | 15 | 16 | 17 | 18 | 19 | 20 | 21 | 22 | 23 | 24 | 25 | 26 | 27 | 28 | 29 | 30 |
|---|---|---|---|---|---|---|---|---|---|---|---|---|---|---|---|---|---|---|---|---|---|---|---|---|---|---|---|---|---|---|